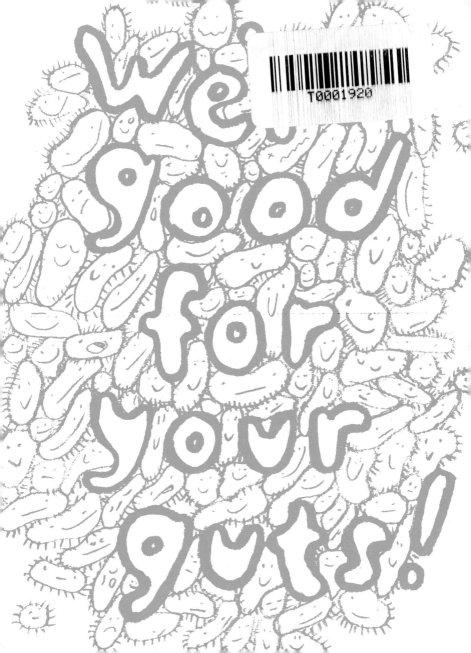

BASIC
FERMENTATION

SANDOR ELLIX KATZ

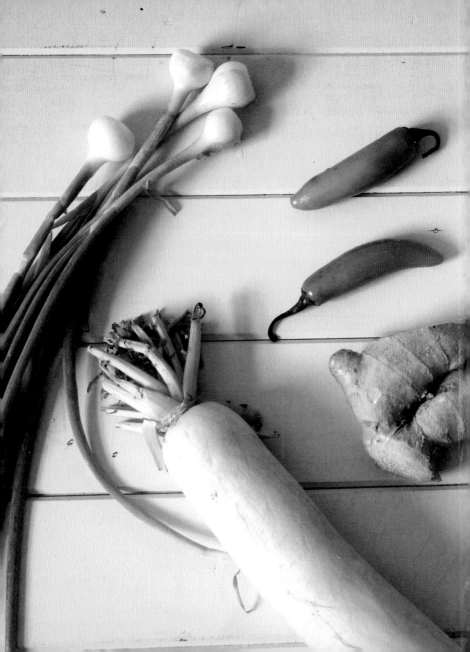

BASIC
FERMENTATION

A DO-IT-YOURSELF GUIDE TO CULTURAL MANIPULATION

WITH ALL NEW PHOTOGRAPHY

SANDOR ELLIX KATZ

MICROCOSM PUBLISHING
PORTLAND, OREGON

BASIC FERMENTATION
A Do-it-yourself Guide to Cultural Manipulation

© Sandor Ellix Katz, 2001, 2017
This edition © Microcosm Publishing, 2011, 2017
First edition, first published 2001
Second edition, first published August 2011
Third edition, first published July 11, 2017

ISBN 978-1-62106-872-3
This is Microcosm #89
Cover illustration by Matt Gauck
Photography and design by Darlene Veenhuizen,
    Pickle Jar Studios, LLC, PickleJarStudios.com
Distributed by PGW and Turnaround in the UK

For a catalog, write or visit:
Microcosm Publishing
2752 N Williams Ave.
Portland, OR 97227
www.microcosmpublishing.com

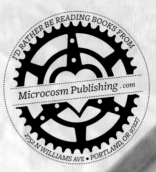

If you bought this on Amazon, that sucks because you could have gotten it cheaper and supported a small independent publisher at MicrocosmPublishing.com

Microcosm Publishing is Portland's most diversified publishing house and distributor with a focus on the colorful, authentic, and empowering. Our books and zines have put your power in your hands since 1996, equipping readers to make positive changes in their lives and in the world around them. Microcosm emphasizes skill-building, showing hidden histories, and fostering creativity through challenging conventional publishing wisdom with books and bookettes about DIY skills, food, bicycling, gender, self-care, and social justice. What was once a distro and record label was started by Joe Biel in his bedroom and has become among the oldest independent publishing houses in Portland, OR. We are a politically moderate, centrist publisher in a world that has inched to the right for the past 80 years.

Global labor conditions are bad, and our roots in industrial Cleveland in the 70s and 80s made us appreciate the need to treat workers right. Therefore, our books are MADE IN THE USA and printed on post-consumer paper.

Library of Congress Cataloging-in-Publication Data

Names: Katz, Sandor Ellix, 1962- author.
Title: Basic fermentation : a do-it-yourself guide to cultural manipulation /
    Sandor Ellix Katz.
Description: Third edition. | Portland, OR : Microcosm Publishing, 2017. |
    Includes bibliographical references.
Identifiers: LCCN 2016035244 (print) | LCCN 2016036007 (ebook) | ISBN
    9781621068723 (pbk.) | ISBN 9781621064466 (epdf) | ISBN 9781621063636
    (epub) | ISBN 9781621062752 (mobi/kindle)
Subjects: LCSH: Fermented foods.
Classification: LCC TP371.44 .K37 2017 (print) | LCC TP371.44 (ebook) | DDC
    664/.024--dc23
LC record available at https://lccn.loc.gov/2016035244

CONTENTS

I originally wrote this short book in 2001. By then I had earned the nickname "Sandorkraut" from friends for my devotion to making and sharing sauerkraut and other fermented delicacies, and I had taught several kraut-making workshops. I first learned to make kraut eight years earlier, in 1993, soon after I moved from my hometown of New York City to a rural community in Tennessee, where I got involved in gardening and cooking for large groups.

Like most people in almost every part of the world, I grew up with flavors of fermentation. As a kid, one of my favorite foods was pickles, juicy cucumbers fermented with garlic and dill, in an Eastern European style. We called them sour pickles and bought them at an old-world deli, and they were infinitely more delicious to me than the vinegar pickles on supermarket shelves. But I didn't know anything about how they were made; I wasn't asking a lot of questions about food back then, just eating. Later I started learning about the immune-stimulating and digestive benefits of these and other live-culture foods. But it wasn't until I had a garden, and an abundance of cabbage, that I had a practical reason to learn how to make it into kraut, and I couldn't quite believe how easy it was. That first kraut was so alive and delicious! It ignited in me a desire to learn more about different realms of fermentation. I learned to make yogurt and country wines, I started a sourdough and learned to bake bread with it. I even learned to make miso that first year.

Over time, I earned a reputation, and friends who were turning their family homestead into an eco-education center, The Sequatchie Valley Institute, invited me to teach my first sauerkraut-making workshop, as part of a larger food skill-sharing event they called Food for Life, in 1998. (As of 2016 Food for Life continues every year.) That first teaching experience taught me that many people project their generalized anxiety about bacteria onto these ancient foods, which have always been prized for their safety. It was challenging, fun, and exciting to be able to demystify fermentation for people. Teaching at Food for Life became an annual tradition that I looked forward to.

In 2001, I decided to spend the summer in Maine, at the home of my dear friend Ed Curran and his wonderful family. My only regret about spending the summer there was missing Food for Life that summer, so I decided to participate from a distance by writing down all my fermentation recipes and sending them in my place. What I produced is this book, though my initial edition was all text, without any images, and self-published at a copy shop. The original self-published zine in the summer of 2001 was called *Wild Fermentation: A Do-It-Yourself Guide to Cultural Manipulation*. Writing it made me realize how much I had to say on the topic of fermentation, and it led me to more extensive experimentation and research, and two longer books: *Wild Fermentation: The Flavor, Nutrition, and Craft of Live-Culture Foods* (2003), and *The Art of Fermentation* (2012). Fermentation education has become my career; I call myself a fermentation revivalist; and I have taught many hundreds of workshops in almost every state and four continents.

As I have traversed the country and the globe teaching (and learning) about fermentation, and promoting the more in-depth books I wrote on the topic, copies of my original zine keep popping up. I had encouraged Microcosm and a few other zine distributors to continue making copies and selling them, and really it contains all the information you need to get started fermenting at home. For many people, a smaller (and cheaper) book is exactly what they want. In 2011, Microcosm asked if they could reformat the original zine, and they published a new edition with attractive graphics and a great pocket-sized format. As it started to show up in online searches, it created some confusion, as it shared a title with my book *Wild Fermentation* (though with different subtitles). With this new expanded edition, filled with clear, full-color instructional photos, we decided to give it a new title, to clear up any confusion. But the text is my original 2001 text, and it remains a perfect introduction to fermentation. Have fun fermenting, don't be afraid to experiment, and if you want to go deeper, check out my later books....

Sandor Ellix Katz
December 2016

❧INTRODUCTION❧

Mix flour and water in a bowl and let it sit on your kitchen counter. Within days it will start to bubble. What is sourdough?

Fermentation happens. It is the path of least resistance. Yeast and bacteria are everywhere, in every breath we take and every bite we eat. Try as you might to eradicate them with antibacterial soaps and antibiotic drugs, there is no escaping them.

These microbial cultures populate our digestive tracts and play a critical role in breaking down the food we eat. They are ubiquitous agents of transformation, feasting upon decaying matter, constantly shifting dynamic life forces from one miraculous and horrible creation to the next. We humans are in a symbiotic relationship with these microscopic living beings. Without them life could not be sustained.

Certain microbial organisms can be harnessed to manifest extraordinary culinary transformations.

Fermentation gives us beer and wine, as well as bread, yogurt, miso, sauerkraut, tempeh and countless other exotic delicacies enjoyed by cultures around the globe. Fermentation is so widespread because it preserves and enhances the foods it alters.

In this book I explain simple methods for a variety of fermented foods. My focus is on basic processes of transformation. These ancient rituals have been conducted for many generations. To me, each ferment is magical and filled with mystery. I am not a scientist intent on distinguishing the microbial agent or identifying the specific enzymatic transformations it causes. Nor am I a technician interested in sterile environments or maintaining exact temperatures. I live deep in the woods, "off the grid," and I cook in a communal kitchen that I share

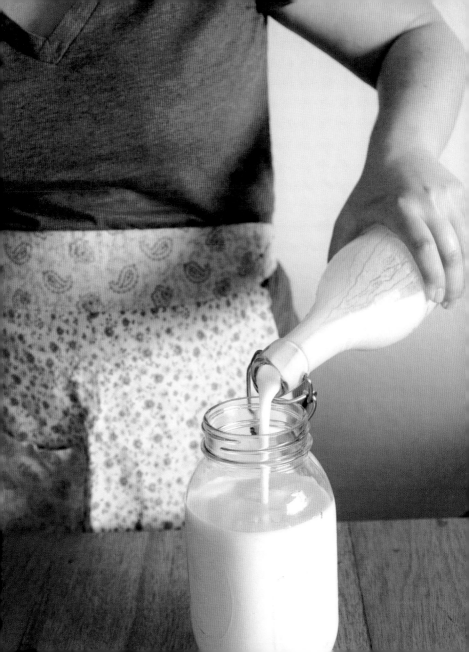

with twenty other people—heated in winter by a wood stove with no thermostat. Though the home brew and wine making books emphasize chemical sterilization and exacting temperature control, all the basic fermented foods predate such technology and can be done low-tech.

Wild fermentation involves creating conditions in which naturally-occurring organisms thrive and proliferate. Wild foods—microbes included—possess great power, some direct unmediated force of the rhythms of the earth. I like to tap into this power by eating weeds—including roots with the soil still clinging to it, hunting for berries and fermenting sauerkraut and sourdough and sour cream. But I also love the fruits of cultivation. I've included several fermentation processes that involve obtaining specific selected cultivated cultures. Each of these came to be out of a wild ferment that occurred in some unique place and set of conditions.

I am writing these techniques down so I can share them with other folks wh like to do it themselves in the kitchen. I am less an expert than a self-taught fetishist. In our kitchen at Short Mountain Sanctuary, bubbling science projects clutter every horizontal surface. Many of the projects are ongoing, as we develop a symbiotic rhythm with these tiny fermenting beings, feeding them regularly so that they feed us regularly.

I am carrying on a long, continuous tradition of nourishing people with good, wholesome food. My father, Joe Katz, a lifelong gardener and the son of a gardener, is endlessly creative at lavishing guests with his garden's bounty; my mother, Rita Ellix, was a lover of fine food who taught me basic culinary skill and aesthetics; my grandmother, Betty Ellix, tirelessly prepared the foods I think of as my cultural heritage. I am proud to be following in their footsteps. I firmly believe that the energy and love we put into food adds infinite nourishing qualities to what we prepare. Nourishment is a path of healing and service, that we can follow and readily share with others.

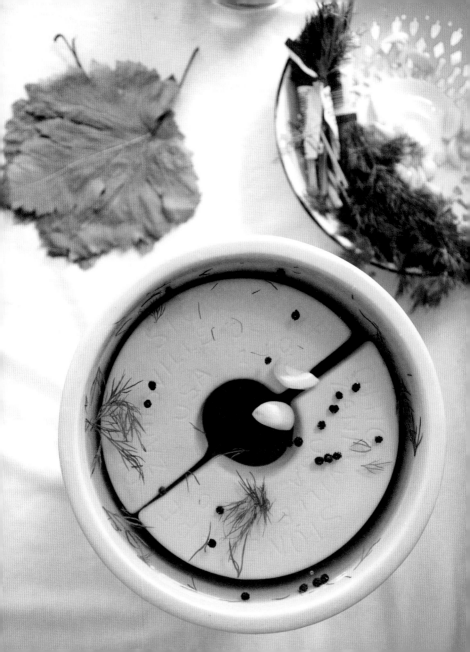

Live, unpasteurized fermented foods have extraordinary nutritional value. They feed the bacteria which broke them down directly into your digestive system, where they keep breaking down food, aiding digestion and nutritional absorption. Nutritional supplement folks call these organisms "probiotic," a play on the word antibiotic, and there is a huge market for probiotic supplements. But whatever a capsule can feed you, a regular variety of live fermented foods can feed you infinitely better. These foods are also abundant in vitamin B-12, which is particularly hard to come by in vegetarian food. But nutritional factoids are extraneous. Taste some miso soup or fresh kraut and your taste buds will tell you that this is something your body needs.

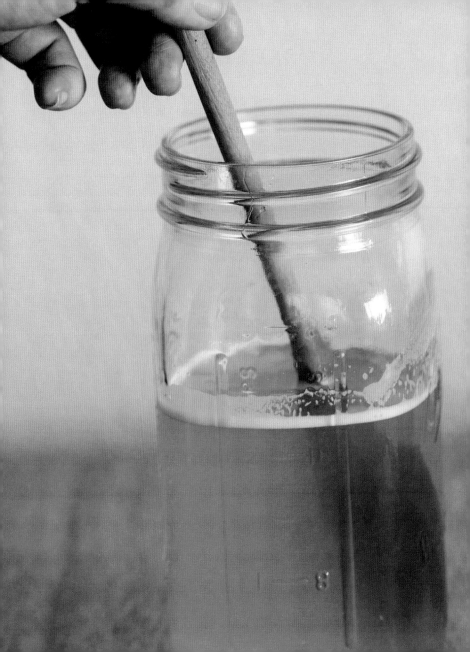

⌁SAUERKRAUT⌁

It all started with sauerkraut. I'd loved it as a kid in New York City, frequently chowing down on street vendor hot dogs, always with mustard and kraut. My dad told me it had been dubbed "liberty cabbage" when he was a kid and the U.S. was at war with the krauts. I also loved it on reuben sandwiches— classically corned beef, thousand island dressing, sauerkraut with cheese melted over it all. When I stopped eating such mysterious and unsavory processed meat products I ended up not eating much sauerkraut.

That is, until I hooked up with macrobiotics, a dietary ideology and practice that I adhered to for a couple of years. The regime is restrictive— mostly grains and vegetables and legumes, prepared in simple ways. Macrobiotics emphasizes the health benefits and in particular the digestive stimulation provided by live, unpasteurized sauerkraut and other brine pickles. I started eating sauerkraut near-daily and have been making crock after crock of the stuff for almost two decades, earning the nickname Sandorkraut.

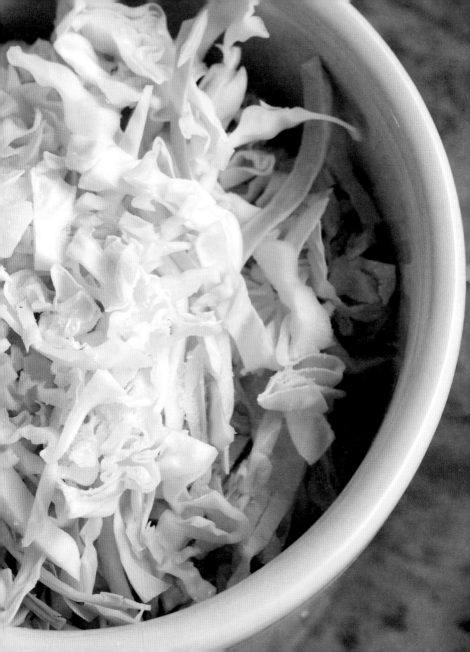

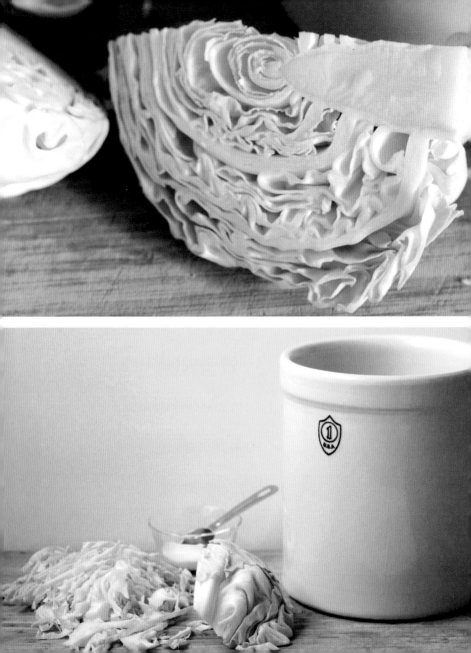

Sauerkraut is easy to make:

INGREDIENTS *for one gallon:*
Cabbage (approximately 5 pounds)
Sea salt (approximately 3 tablespoons)

SPECIAL EQUIPMENT:
Ceramic crock or food-grade plastic bucket—cylindrical shape is what's important.
Plate that fits inside crock or bucket.
One gallon jug filled with water
Cloth cover

PROCESS:
Chop or grate cabbage, finely or coarsely, with or without hearts, however you like it. I love to mix green and red cabbage to end up with bright pink kraut.

Sprinkle salt on the cabbage as you chop it. The salt makes the cabbage sweat, and this creates the brine (salty water) in which the cabbage can ferment and sour without rotting. Do not use iodized salt because iodine inhibits bacterial action.

Three tablespoons of salt is a rough average. According to the food scientists, the sauerkraut process works best in 2-3% brine solution. I never measure the salt, I just shake some on after I chop up each quarter cabbage. I use more salt in the summer, less in the winter. It is possible to make kraut without salt, using ground kelp and other sea vegetables instead.

Add other vegetables (onions, garlic, other greens, brussels sprouts, small whole heads of cabbage, whatever) and herbs and spices (caraway seeds, dill seeds, anything) as you like. Experiment.

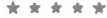

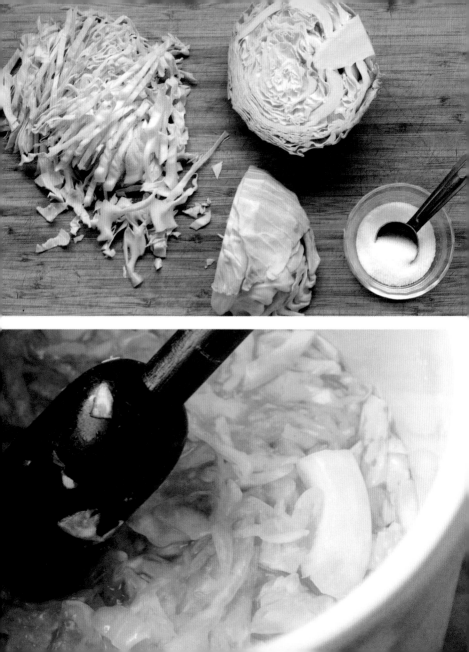

Mix ingredients together and *pack into crock*. Pack just a bit into the crock at a time and tamp it down hard using your fists or any sturdy kitchen implement. The tamping packs the kraut tight in the crock and helps force water out of the cabbage.

Cover kraut with a plate or some other lid that fits snugly inside the crock. Place a clean weight, like a gallon jug filled with water, on the cover. This weight is what will keep the cabbage submerged in the brine. Cover the whole thing with a cloth or pillow case to keep dust and flies out.

Press down on the weight periodically until the brine rises above the cover. This can take a while, as the salt slowly draws water out of the cabbage. Some cabbage, particularly if it is old, simply contains less water. If for some reason the brine does not rise above the plate level by the next day, add enough salt water to bring the brine level above the plate.

Check the kraut after a few days. If any moldy scum appears on the surface, scrape it away. Taste the kraut. It should start to be tangy after a few days, and the taste gets stronger as time passes. In cool temperatures, kraut can keep improving for months and months. Eventually it becomes soft and the flavor turns less pleasant. The process is faster in summer, slower in winter.

Enjoy. Scoop out a bowlful at a time and keep it in the fridge. I start when the kraut is young and enjoy its evolving flavor over the course of a few weeks. Try the sauerkraut juice that will be left in the bowl after the kraut is eaten: sauerkraut juice is a rare delicacy and unparalleled digestive tonic.

Each time you scoop some kraut out of the crock, you have to repack it carefully. Make sure the kraut is packed tight in the crock, the surface is level, and the cover and weight are clean. Sometimes brine evaporates, so if the kraut is not submerged below brine just add salted water as necessary.

★ ★ ★ ★ ★ ★ ★ ★ ★ ★

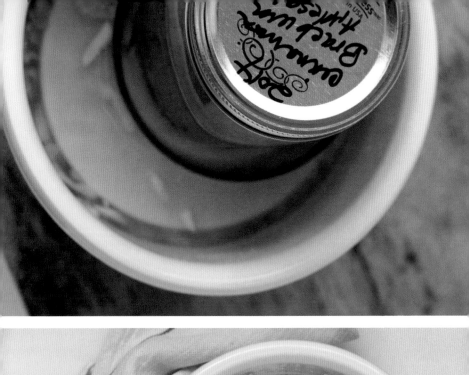

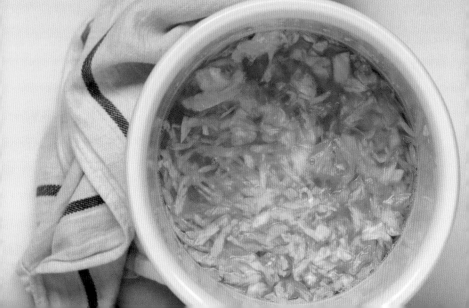

Some people preserve kraut by canning and heat-processing it. This can be done, but so much of the power of sauerkraut is its aliveness that I wonder: why kill it?

Develop a rhythm: Start a new batch before the previous batch runs out. I take what remains in the crock out, pack the crock with fresh salted cabbage, then pour the old kraut and its juices over the new kraut. This gives the new batch a boost with an active culture starter.

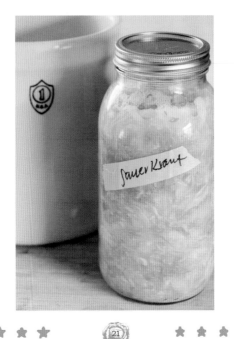

While researching this book, I found a lab project for a food sciences class at the University of Wisconsin where they make kraut and analyze it at intervals during its fermentation period of five weeks at 70 degrees fahrenheit. What was interesting to me is that the process involves a succession of microorganisms. According to the experiment's write-up:

"As no starter cultures are added to the system, this is referred to as a wild fermentation. The normal flora of the cabbage leaves is relied upon to include the organisms responsible for a desirable fermentation, one that will enhance preservation and organoleptic acceptability. The floral succession is governed mainly by the pH of the growth medium. Initially, a coliform starts the fermentation. Coliforms which have contributed to our lab-made sauerkraut in recent years have included *Klebsiella pneumoniac, K. oxcytoca* and *Enterobacter cloacae*. As acid is produced, an environment more favorable for *Leuconostoc* is quickly formed. The coliform population declines as the population of a strain of *Leuconostoc* is a heterofermentative lactic acid bacterium, much gas (carbon dioxide) accompanies the acid production during this stage. The pH continues to drop, and a strain of *Lactobacillus* succeeds the *Leuconostoc* (on occasion a strain of *Pediococcus* arises instead of *Lactobacillus*). The complete fermentation, then, involves a succession of three major groups or genera of bacteria, a succession governed by the decreasing pH."

—From John Lindquist, Department of Bacteriology, University of Wisconsin-Madison

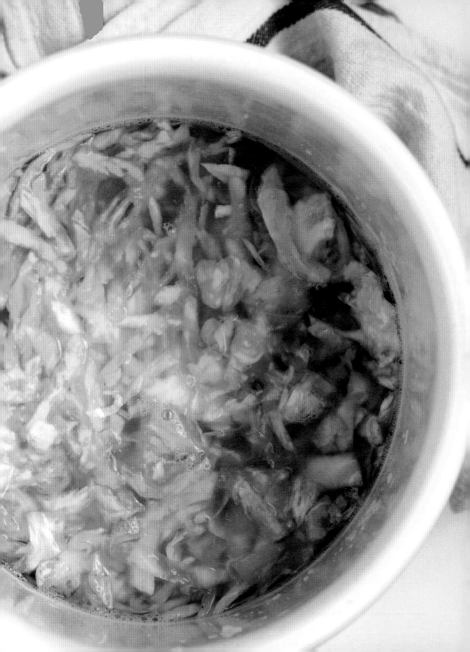

♔ **MISO** ♕

Miso is a uniquely grounding food, the product of a year or more of fermentation. It was noted in the wake of the Hiroshima and Nagasaki nuclear bombings that miso helped survivors of the fallout reduce levels of radiation and heavy metals in their bodies. In our radioactive world we could all do with some healing. Making miso requires great patience, but waiting is the hardest part of the process. Making it is simple. I recommend making and decanting this hearty food in winter.

INGREDIENTS *for one gallon:*
4 cups dried beans
5 cups koji (rice inoculated with spores of *Aspergillus oryzae*, source info below)
1 cup sea salt
2 tablespoons unpasteurized seed miso

SPECIAL EQUIPMENT:
Ceramic crock or food grade plastic bucket
Lid that fits snugly inside (plate or hardwood)
Heavy rock or other weight

PROCESS: *Soak* overnight and *cook until soft* 4 cups of dry beans. Soybeans are classic, but I've used chickpeas, black beans, split peas, lentils, black-eyed peas and more. Cook until the beans are soft and crush easily. Take care not to burn the beans, especially if you're using soybeans, which take a long while to cook.

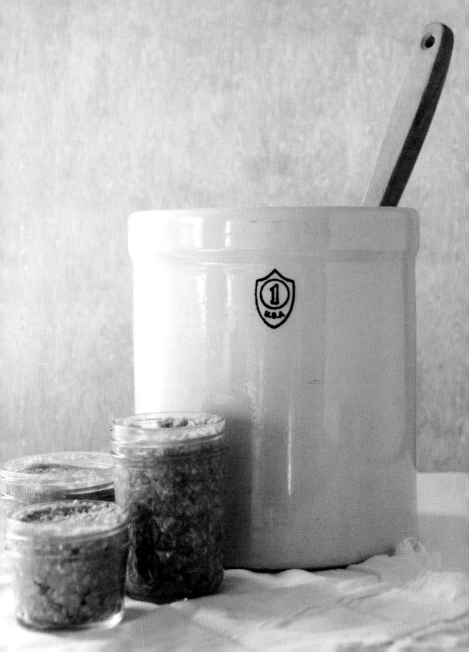

Clean all utensils thoroughly with hot water before you use them. Place a colander over a pot and **drain beans**, reserving bean cooking liquid, covered to keep it warm.

Mash beans to desired smoothness, using a potato masher, ricer, grain mill, food processor, whatever tools are available. I generally use a potato masher and leave the beans fairly chunky.

Take about 3 cups of the reserved bean cooking liquid (or hot water if there isn't enough or you accidentally poured it down the drain) and mix into the salt and seed miso. After that is well mixed, add the koji. Finally add this mixture to the mashed beans and mix until the texture is uniform. If it seems thicker than miso you've had, add some more bean cooking liquid or hot water to desired consistency. This is your miso; the remaining steps are packaging.

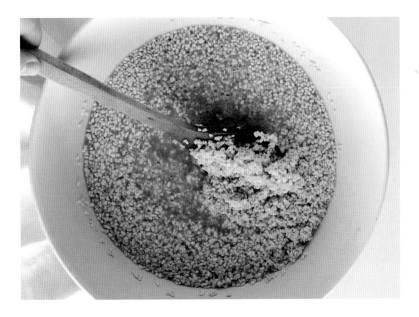

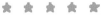

Salt bottom and side surfaces of your fermenting vessel with wet fingers dipped in sea salt. The idea is to have higher salt content at the edges where contaminating bacteria could access the miso.

Pack miso tightly into the crock, taking care to expel air pockets. Smooth the top and sprinkle a layer of salt over it.

Cover with a lid. A hardwood lid cut to exactly the size and shape of the crock is ideal, but I often use the biggest plate I can find that fits inside the crock. Rest a heavy weight on the lid. I find a rock, scrub it clean and boil it. The weight is important because, as with sauerkraut, it forces the solid ferment under the protection of the salty brine. Finally place an outer cover over the whole thing, to keep dust and flies out. Cloth or plastic work well, tied or taped to the crock.

Label clearly with indelible markers. This is important once you have multiple batches going from different years. Store in a cellar, barn or other unheated environment.

Wait. Try some the fall/winter after the first summer of fermentation. Repack it carefully, lightly salting the new top layer. Then try it a year later, even a year after that. The flavor of miso will mellow and develop over time. I tried some nine year-old miso and it was sublime, like a well-aged wine.

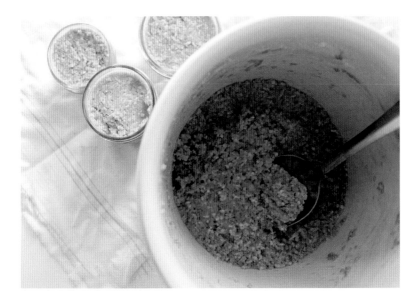

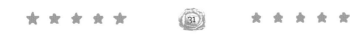

A note on decanting: When you open a crock of miso which has been fermenting for a couple years, the top layer may be quite ugly and off-putting. Skim it off, throw it in the compost, and trust that below the surface the miso will be gorgeous and smell and taste great. I pack miso into thoroughly clean glass jars. If the tops are metal, I use a layer of wax paper between the jar and the lid, as miso causes metal to corrode. I store the jars in the basement. Since fermentation continues, the jars build up pressure, which needs to be periodically released by opening the jars. To avoid that, you can store miso in the fridge.

A note on a cooking with miso: Boiling miso will kill it. When making soups or sauces, cook your stock and just prior to serving turn off the heat, take a little hot liquid out, mix it with miso, return it to the soup, and stir well.

Where to Find Koji

Check with local commercial miso manufacturers to see if they'll sell you koji. The best source I've found is South River Miso Co., Conway, MA 01341, telephone (413) 369-4057, www.southrivermiso.com

They sell koji for $16 per pound. You can make your own koji by inoculating rice with spores of *Aspergillus oryzae*. There are detailed instructions in *The Book of Miso*, listed in the bibliography section.

⌒AMAZAKE⌒

When I make miso each winter, I try to order a little extra rice koji so I can make amazake. Amazake is a particularly dramatic ferment, because in a matter of hours it transforms the starch of plain brown rice into sugars. The result is a uniquely sweet rice porridge, which can be eaten as a pudding, strained into a drink, or used as a bubbly base for pancake batter or bread. Amazake is from Japan, and can be found in refrigerator or freezer sections of many health food stores.

INGREDIENTS *for a half gallon:*
2 cups brown rice
5 cups water
2 cups rice koji

SPECIAL EQUIPMENT:
Half gallon jar
Insulated cooler

PROCESS:
Bring rice and water to a boil. Cook, covered, for 45 minutes, or until most of the water has absorbed. The high proportion of water will result in a somewhat wet batch of rice, which is what you want. Alternatively you can use leftover rice, rehydrating it and warming it by adding boiling water gradually in a pan over a low heat, while breaking up clumps of rice with a spoon or spatula.

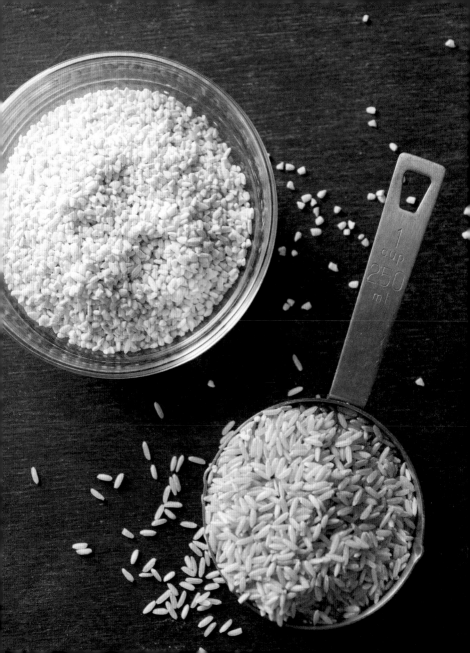

Allow rice to cool, stirring periodically to release heat from the center, until rice is still warm but comfortable to the touch.

Preheat half gallon jar and insulated cooler with hot water.

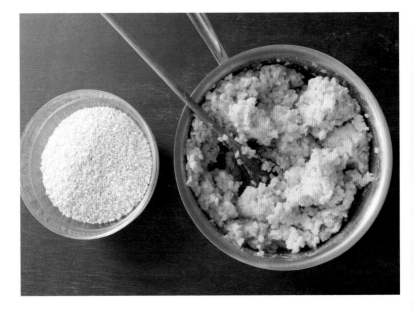

Add koji to warm rice, mix until distribution seems even, and fill preheated jar with the mixture. Cover jar with a piece of cloth and a rubber band, or loosely cap.

Place the jar in the preheated insulated cooler. If much space remains in the cooler, fill it with bottles of hot water— but not too hot to touch— and/or towels. Close the cooler.

Taste the amazake after eight hours. If it is sweet it is ready. If not, rewarm by sitting the jar of amazake in hot water. Being too hot to touch is okay now since you are trying to raise the temperature of the ferment. Re-insulate it for up to eight more hours.

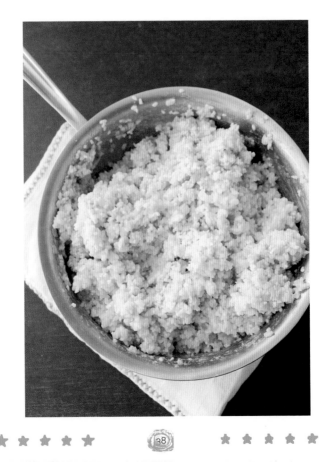

Eat the amazake fresh, either warm or cold. I like its distinctive flavor plain, but I have also enjoyed it seasoned with grated ginger, toasted almonds, and vanilla.

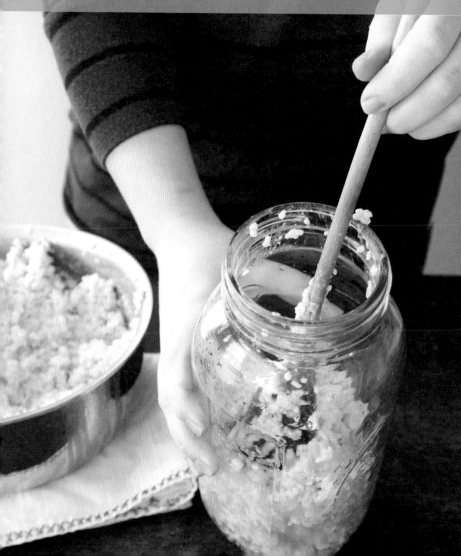

If you plan to store the amazake beyond a couple of hours *bring it to a boil* to stop fermentation before refrigerating. The sweet phase passes rather quickly and the amazake begins to transform into an alcoholic grog, which I understand to be the basis for sake, the delicious and strong Japanese rice wine, though I have never taken the process that far.

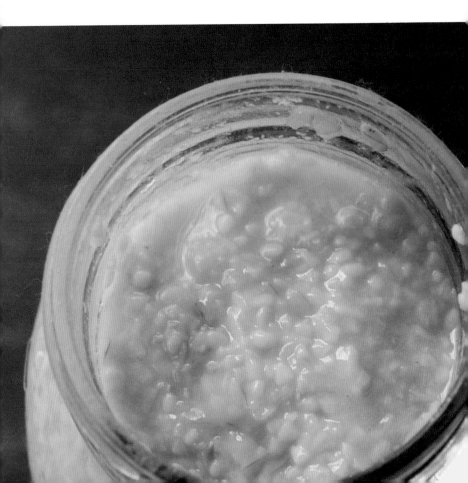

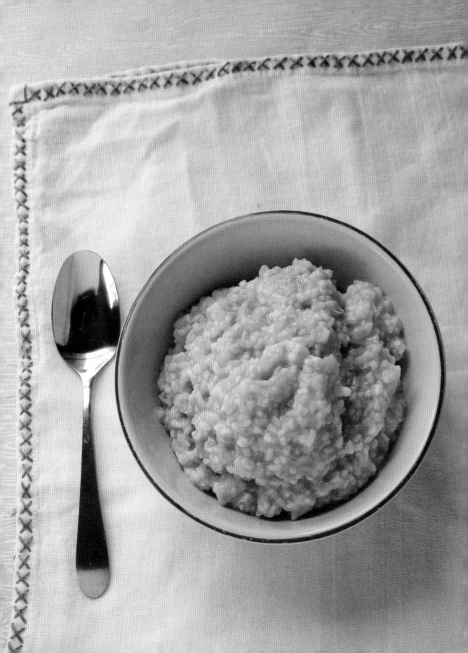

✂SOURDOUGH BREAD✂

Bread is a staple food in many cultures around the world. It can be made from different grains and in an extraordinary variety of style. Many excellent books are devoted exclusively to the fine and nuanced art of bread baking. Bakers I have known feel that bread making is a spiritual exercise that connects them to the life force. I quite agree; like any ferment, bread requires the harnessing and gentle cultivation of life forces, in the form of yeast. Bread also requires the full body involvement of kneading. Kneading develops gluten, the rubbery component of wheat and other grains, which enables the dough to trap bubbles of gas released by the yeast as it reproduces, thus yielding a light and airy loaf of bread.

I will walk you through the most basic sourdough process. I never measure anything when I make bread—I find appropriate proportions through texture. But I have tried to offer rough measurements. Take them with a grain or two of salt. Consider the descriptions of consistency and texture more closely than my somewhat arbitrary quantifications. It takes several days for the yeast to colonize your batter. But once it does you can make bread from it for years, even pass it down unto the generations, the way people used to do these things. Once you experience the magic of sourdough bread making you are likely to want to experiment. Deviate, explore, enjoy!

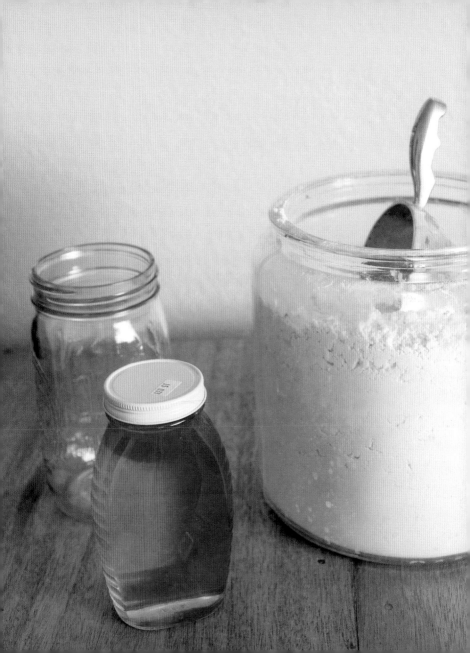

MAKING THE STARTER:

In a quart size jar, *mix* two cups of warm—bath temperature—*water* with four tablespoons of *honey and/or molasses* and one cup of flour. Honey and molasses have very different flavors, but in this process they both serve the same purpose of attracting and stimulating yeast. Likewise, any kind of flour will do. *Stir the mixture vigorously* and cover it with cheesecloth or other porous material that allows free air circulation.

Wait. The batter will attract yeast from the air. Store your batter in a warm place with good air circulation. 70 to 80 degrees Fahrenheit is ideal, but work with what you have. Visit your batter as often as you think of it—at least daily—and stir it vigorously. The more agitation it has the greater exposure it receives to the yeast that will transform it.

After some number of days you will notice *tiny bubbles* releasing at the surface of the batter. That is how you can tell the yeast is active. Note that the action of stirring the batter may create some bubbles. Do not confuse these with the bubbles the batter produces when you are not actively introducing air into the mixture. The number of days it will take for yeast to colonize your batter will depend on environmental factors. Every ecosystem has its own unique yeast populations. This is why sourdoughs from specific locations can be so distinctive.

Many cookbooks recommend to start a sourdough with a pinch of packaged yeast to get the process going more quickly. I prefer the gratifying purity of the yeast magically finding its way to the dough. If you do not find bubbles forming after three or four days, find a warmer spot or add a pinch of packaged yeast.

Add a little *more flour* (roughly a quarter cup) to the mixture each day and continue stirring for three or four days after the bubbles first appear. You can add any kind of flour, or leftover cooked grains, or rolled oats or whole millet or other whole grains soaked in water overnight. You are feeding the sourdough.

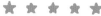

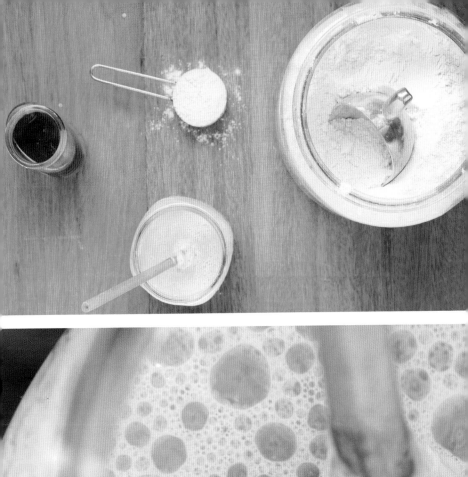

The batter will get thicker, and start to rise, or hold some of the gas the yeast releases, but you want it to remain essentially liquid in form. Add more water if the sourdough gets so thick that it starts to become solid. Once you have a thick bubbly batter *pour half of it into a mixing bowl.* This will become your bread to bake (see below); *the half in the jar is your "starter"* to keep the sourdough going.

Add water roughly equal to the volume you removed for bread, and some more flour. *Keep it going* by feeding it a little flour every day or two if you are baking at least weekly. If you use it less frequently you can refrigerate it (thus slowing the yeast) and feed it about once a week, then take it out of the fridge and feed it a day or two before you plan to bake to warm it up and get the yeast active again.

MAKING BREAD FROM THE STARTER:

Now, back to the batter in the bowl: Add a cup of water and enough flour or leftover cooked grains, rolled oats, whole millet or other soaked whole grains to *make it a thick batter again.* Stir it well. Let it sit in a warm place, covered with a towel or cloth, for about 8 to 24 hours, stirring occasionally, until it is good and bubbly.

When it is good and bubbly, *add more flour and a little salt.* Salt inhibits the yeast, which is why we don't add it early in the process. But bread without salt tastes flat and lacking.

Let it sit, covered, in a warm place for a few hours till it increases noticeably in bulk. Gradually add flour, stir well, and let the dough rise, until it becomes so thick you cannot stir it with a spoon.

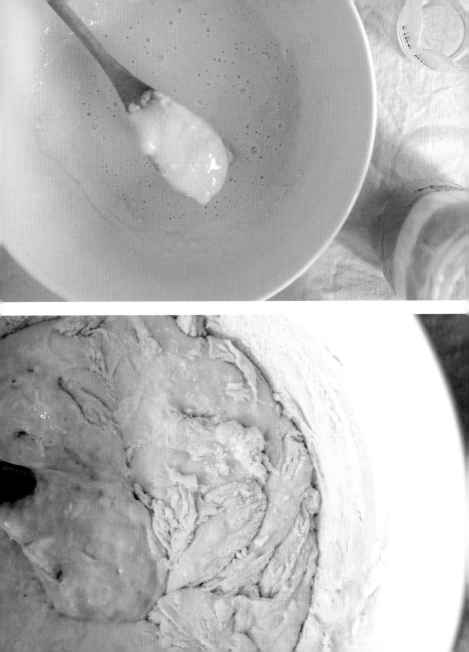

Knead the dough well on a floured surface. If you have never kneaded this involves pushing the heel of your palm into the dough, stretching and flattening it, then folding an edge into the center, pushing and stretching with the palm of your hand, then folding another edge into the center, etc. As you knead, you may need to sprinkle additional flour onto the dough and the kneading surface if the dough starts to feel sticky, which it can as the flour absorbs the moisture of the dough. On the other hand, if you add too much flour the dough and resulting bread can be overly dense. You need to knead long enough to "work the gluten" so the dough develops elasticity. Give it at least 10-15 minutes. A good way to tell if you've kneaded enough is to poke a finger into the dough and remove it. Well-kneaded elastic dough should resist the indentation and push back toward its original form.

Place the kneaded ball of dough into a clean, lightly-oiled bowl. Cover with a moist warm towel and set the bowl in a warm place for the dough to rise. *Rise* the dough until it roughly doubles in bulk, anywhere from one to many hours, depending on the temperature and the character of the dough and yeast that has developed. Once it has doubled, punch it down and *form into loaves*, kneading each loaf for a moment, sprinkling just a little more flour if the dough is sticky, and place loaves in lightly-oiled loaf pans.

Rise for another hour or so, until the loaves have risen substantially. Then preheat oven to 400 degrees, and *bake.*

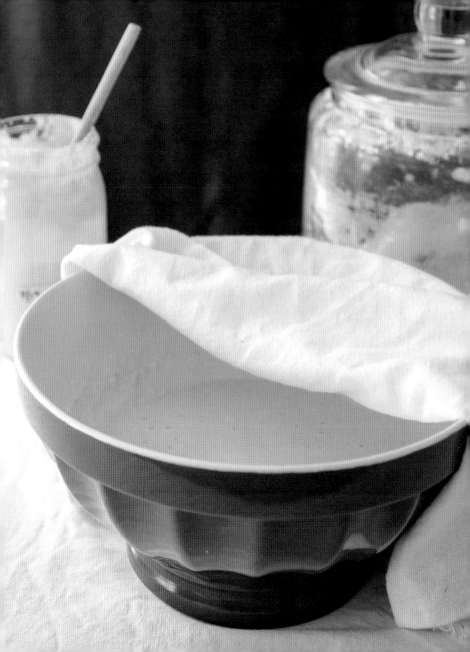

Check loaves after 30 minutes. Most likely, unless they are primarily white flour and extremely light, or small loaves, they will require more time than this—maybe 35 minutes, maybe an hour, maybe even more. To *test doneness* of the bread, remove it upside down from the loaf pan. Tap the bottom of the loaf. When it is done it will sound hollow, like a drum. If it's not done, return it to the oven quickly.

When the bread is done, remove it from the hot pan and cool it on a rack or cool surface.

The bread continues to cook and set as it cools. It's hard to *be patient* when it smells so good, but try to wait ten minutes and it'll taste that much better

This is the basic process. From here, using your sourdough starter, the possibilities are endless. Try any kind of flour. Incorporate cooked grains, or whole grains soaked overnight. Use milk or soy milk or dairy ferments or amazake instead of water. Add savory herbs or raisins and nuts. Add miso. Bread is infinite.

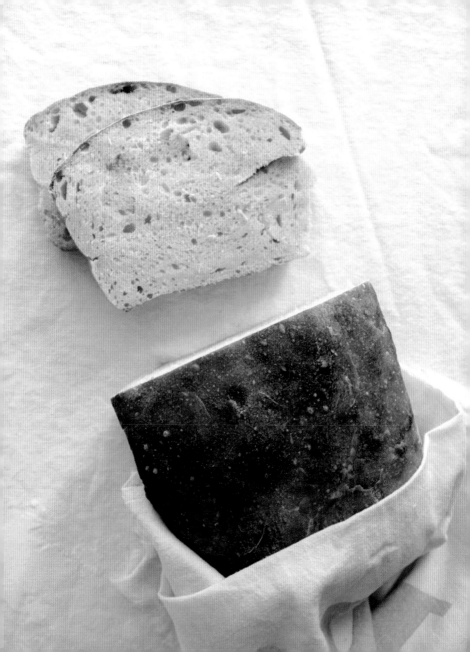

☞INJERA☜

One type of sourdough bread is injera—a spongy bread that is a staple in Ethiopian cuisine. In Ethiopian restaurants, food is served on trays lined with injera, and you eat by ripping off pieces of injera and scooping food into it. Any saucy dish would be good on injera and an internet search will yield many yummy Ethiopian recipes. Injera is generally cooked in advance and served at a room temperature.

INGREDIENTS:
2 cups flour (teff is the grain used in Ethiopia; use some of that if you can find it, along with wheat or other grains)
2 ½ cups water
Sourdough starter (optional)
1 tsp baking powder
1 tsp salt
vegetable oil (I use canola)

PROCESS:
Mix flour and water in bowl (glass or ceramic, not metal). If you have sourdough starter, use less flour and water and add them to your starter. Stir well. The mixture should have the consistency of thin pancake batter. Add more water if necessary. Cover with cheesecloth.
Leave to ferment in a warm place, stirring as often as you think of it.

If you began with an active starter, leave it for about 24 hours; if you're starting from scratch it will likely take three days. When it's ready it will be bubbly.

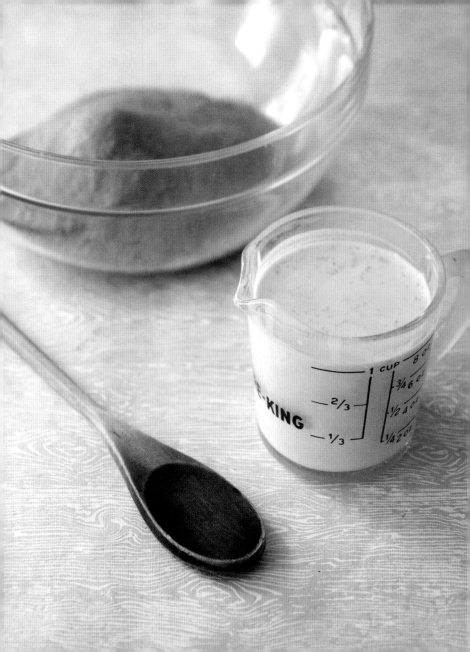

When you are ready to cook injeras, *add baking powder and salt* and stir well. Let the mixture sit for a few moments before cooking.

The baking powder makes the injera extra bubbly and spongy.

If you're trying to be a purist, skip the baking powder if your batter is good and bubbly.

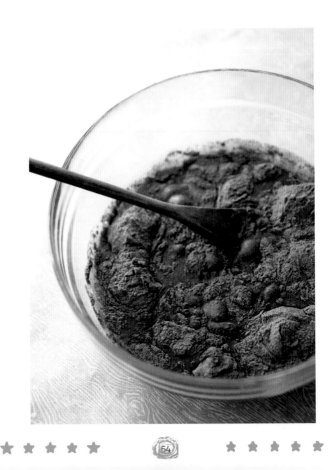

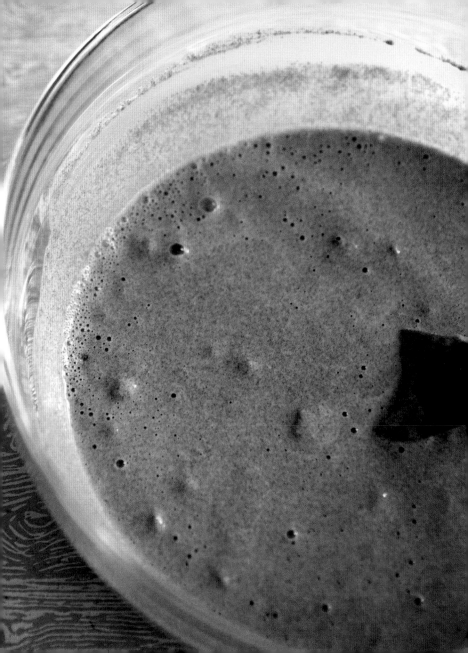

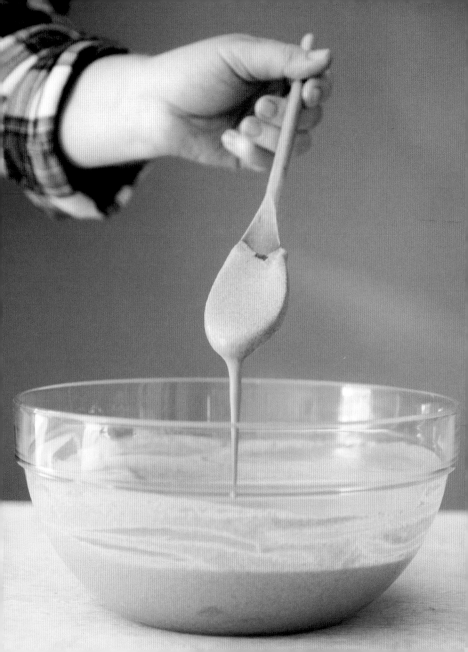

Heat a well-seasoned cast-iron skillet (or anything you would make pancakes on) over medium heat. Brush on or otherwise lightly coat pan with oil.

Pour batter onto hot skillet, taking care to spread it as thinly as possible. If batter won't spread thinly, thin it with a little more water.

Cook until holes appear all over and the top is dry. *Cook on one side only*; do not flip. Remove from pan onto towel to cool.

Cooled injera may be *stacked and wrapped* in a towel.

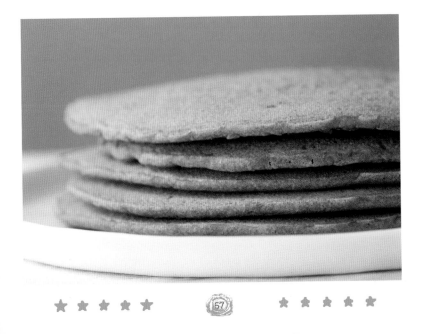

⌇ETHIOPIAN HONEY WINE⌇

I got into beer and wine-making for a while, but the methods I learned involved numerous complex steps and rigorous sterilization, which turned me off. I especially hated the idea of killing the wild yeast present on the skins of fruit to assure the success of a particular proven strain of yeast. One great and different beer-making book, Stephen Harrod Buhner's *Sacred and Healing Beers: The Secrets of Ancient Fermentation* (see bibliography) refers to this emphasis in the literature as "Teutonic."

Alcoholic ferments—beers, wines, meads—are ancient and widespread. When I spent a few months traveling in Africa in the mid-1980s, almost every village had some kind of local ferment to offer, often palm wines bubbling away in gourds. I knew simple, quick, delicious bottle-free wines were possible, and I was ecstatic when I came across a recipe for T'ej, Ethiopian honey wine, in a cookbook that I only saw once and can't even remember the name of. But I followed these basic proportions and steps and have made many excellent sweet honey wines. This wine complements the injera (above) quite perfectly and could inspire you to have an Ethiopian feast.

INGREDIENTS:
2 cups honey (raw and unfiltered if available)
Half gallon of water
1 cup dried hops flowers

SPECIAL EQUIPMENT:
1 gallon ceramic crock or wide-mouth jar
1 gallon glass jug (the kind you can buy apple juice in)
Airlock (from wine supply shop, under $1)

PROCESS:
Mix water and honey in the crock or jar. Cover with a towel or cloth and set aside in a warm room for three days.

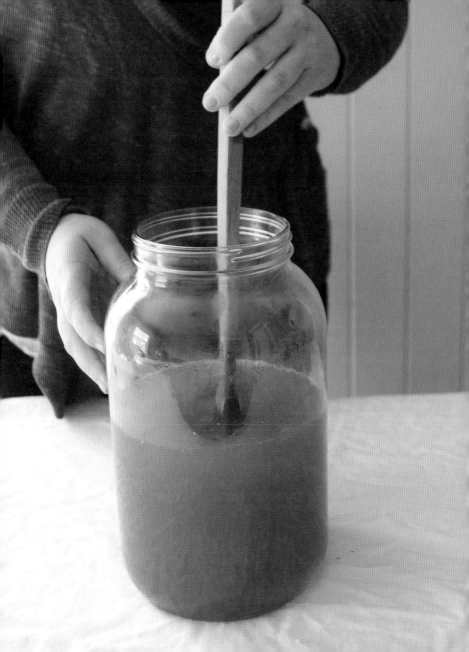

After three or more days, take out two cups of the honey water and bring it to a boil. Steep half the hops in the hot honey water, until cool. Then add the hops-steeped honey water and the hops you didn't add to the hot water to the crock or jar of honey water. The reason for this is to extract the hops flavor by steeping it in hot water, but also to capture some of the yeast on the dried hops leaves without killing it.

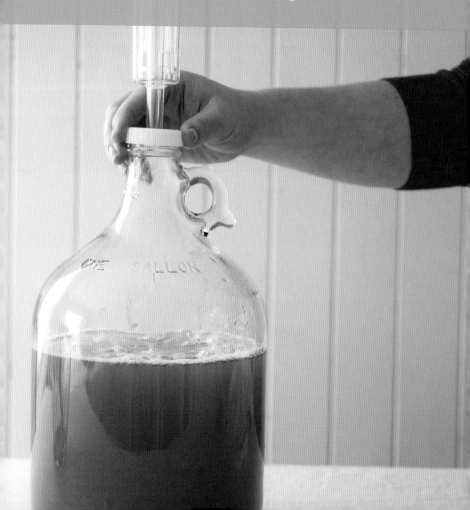

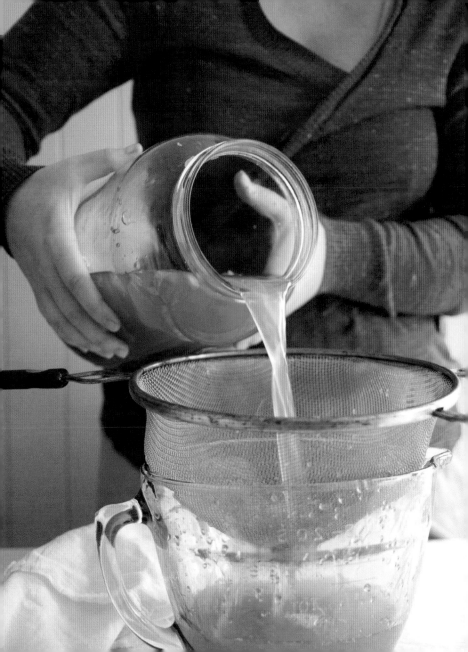

At this point you can **add other flavorings** as well. My favorite was adding ground coffee beans. I've also added bananas, lemons, berries, and a number of different herbs. *Stir daily.* It should be bubbly and fragrant.

Taste your wine frequently to see how it progresses. After about five days *strain out solid ingredients* and transfer wine into a clean one gallon glass jug. If the jug is not full, you can add water and honey in 4:1 ratio to fill.

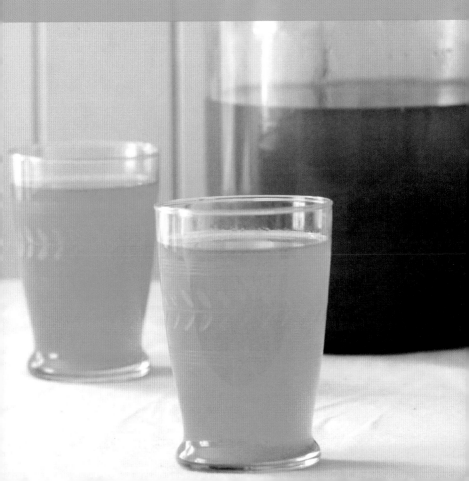

Leave for about two weeks, until bubbling slows. This is "instant" gratification wine. Drink it when it is ready, or bottle it for short-term storage; I have not had great results aging it.

If you wish to explore beer or winemaking more in depth, bookstores and beer/winemaking supply shops are full of books to guide you. Information on the *Sacred and Healing Herbal Beers* I refer to above can be found in the bibliography at the end of this booklet.

✒VINEGAR✒

The simplest vinegar is wine gone bad. If you leave your T'ej (above) in the crock, eventually it will become vinegar.

Here is the basic process for making cider vinegar:

Pour *apple cider*—raw and unfiltered if at all possible—but without any preservative chemicals that could kill our little friends who make this transformation possible—into a crock or wide-mouth bottle, covered with cheesecloth.

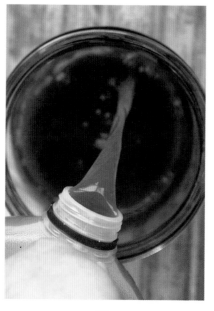

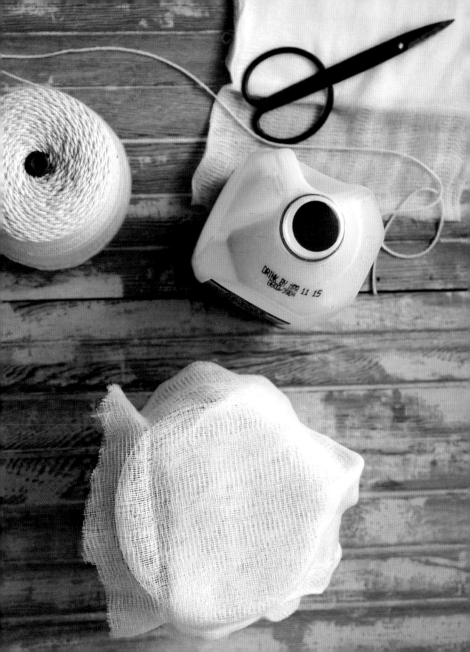

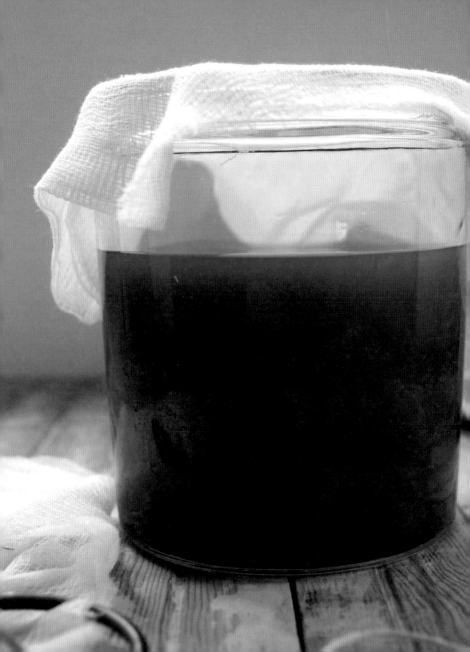

Store at room temperature. *Stir and taste daily*, noting the development of an alcoholic and then vinegary taste. The full process takes about four weeks, depending on temperature and your environment, and will leave a "mother" in the vinegar, which can be used as a starter for future batches of vinegar.

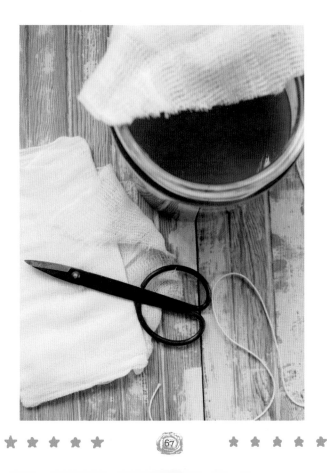

✑YOGURT✑

No cultured food is better known or acknowledged for its health benefits than yogurt. Yogurt is delicious and easy to make. Yogurt is an extremely versatile food that can be enjoyed savory as well as sweet. Your digestive tract will be grateful for an abundant and frequent supply of yogurt.

INGREDIENTS *for half gallon of yogurt:*
Half gallon minus a half cup (60 oz.) of milk or soy milk
Half a cup of fresh live culture yogurt for starter (soy milk yogurt is available in health food stores)

SPECIAL EQUIPMENT:
Half gallon jar
Insulated cooler

PROCESS:
Preheat half gallon jar and insulated cooler with hot water. Heat milk to the point where it feels hot but it is not hard to keep your (clean!) finger in it. Or use a thermometer to heat milk to 110 degrees Fahrenheit. I do not pasteurize milk first because I make yogurt out of fresh raw goat milk and am interested in maintaining the live cultures present in the milk. Many people heat the milk to a boil before making yogurt. If you do that, which can produce a thicker yogurt, take care to stir frequently while you heat the milk to avoid burning it. Cool the milk as quickly as possible by setting the pot with the hot milk into bowls or pots of cold water, until you can place a finger in it.

Mix starter yogurt into the hot milk. Stir well and pour mixture into the pre-heated jar, loosely capped.

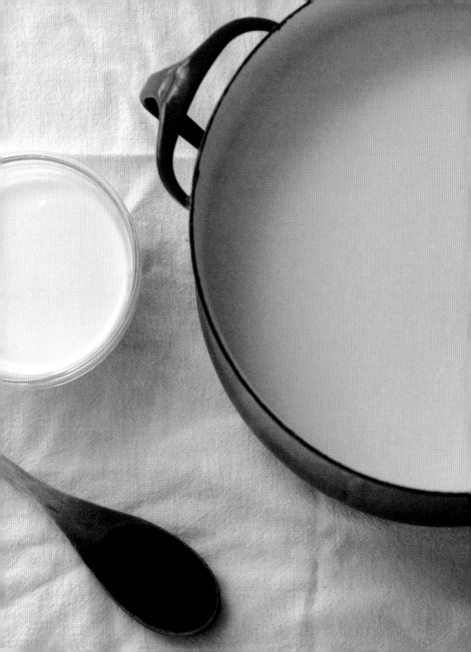

Place the jar in the preheated insulated cooler. If much space remains in the cooler, fill it with bottles of hot water (not too hot to touch) and/or towels. Close the cooler. Place the cooler in a warm spot.

Check the yogurt after 8-12 hours. It should have a tangy flavor and some thickness. Thickness will vary with the unique cultural and environmental conditions.

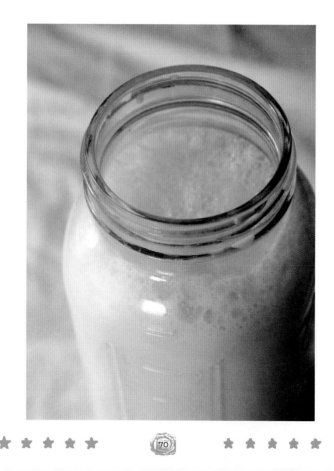

Yogurt can store in the refrigerator for weeks. *Save some of your yogurt to use as starter* in the next batch. If after a number of generations your yogurt culture seems to be weakening, freshen it by introducing some new starter yogurt.

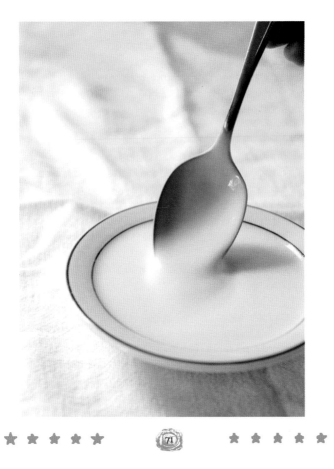

✋TARA AND KEFIR✋

DAIRY RELATED FERMENTS

I recently attended a workshop with my weed-eating guru Susun Weed, author of *Healing Wise* and several other great herbals. She served us delicious homemade goat cheese from her goats, and I told her about our goats. We bonded, talking about making yogurt and cheese. When I left, she gave me a plastic bag containing curds of a culture she likes to use in goats milk, that she calls Tara.

Susun was given Tara by some Tibetan monk friends, who brought the culture from Tibet. I wasn't at home with fresh goats milk when I got the culture, so I just mixed it with store-bought whole milk and left it in a jar at room temperature for about 24 hours. I love the sweet fizzy light drink it produces.

Tara is the Tibetan cousin of the ferment more widely known as Kefir, which originates in the Central Asian region called the Caucasus. A product called Kefir is sold in health food stores, but this bears little resemblance to the version you can make at home with "grains," actually colonies of yeast and bacteria that look like curds, which you strain out of the milk after fermentation, then use to start the next batch. Kefir is especially easy to make because it requires no temperature control and takes just a day. The hard part would be coming by the grains to get started, but there are online groups of kefir enthusiasts eager to provide grains to new converts.

Here's how easy it is to make:

Fill a jar with milk, no more than two-thirds full, and *add your kefir grains*. Tighten the cap if you want your kefir fizzy, leave it loose if not. For people who do not drink milk, this same process can be done with soy or rice or nut milk or juice or honey water.

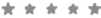

Leave at room temperature for about 24 hours, agitating the jar periodically. Strain out grains.

Enjoy your kefir, keep in the refrigerator, and use grains for another batch. Grains can stay in the fridge in milk (or alternative medium) for a couple of weeks, or can be frozen for a couple of months or dried for a couple of years.

✲BUTTERMILK✲

Buttermilk is great for pancakes, biscuits, and other baking projects. A little commercial live culture buttermilk can be added to plain milk, left at room temperature for about twenty-four hours, and it's all buttermilk, which can be stored in a refrigerator for months.

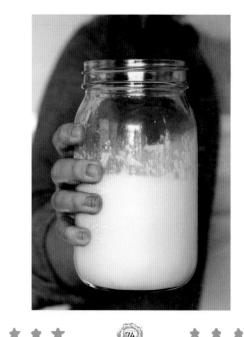

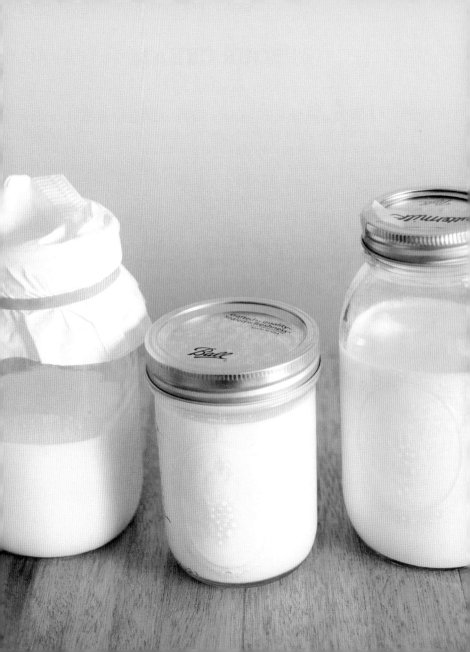

❦ SOUR CREAM ❧

When we run out of refrigerator space for our fresh goats milk, or if I'm feeling too lazy to make cheese, I just leave a gallon of milk on the kitchen counter, with the cap loose. Bacteria present in the milk or in the air, will, after a few days, convert enough lactose to lactic acid that the milk separates. Skim the cream off the top and boy is it sour! Some people find its flavor to be so strong as to be unpleasant, but to me it is delicious and extreme sour cream.

You can do this with yogurt or kefir, as well. Leaving these ferments at room temperature to curdle themselves can produce cheeses with excellent flavors and textures.

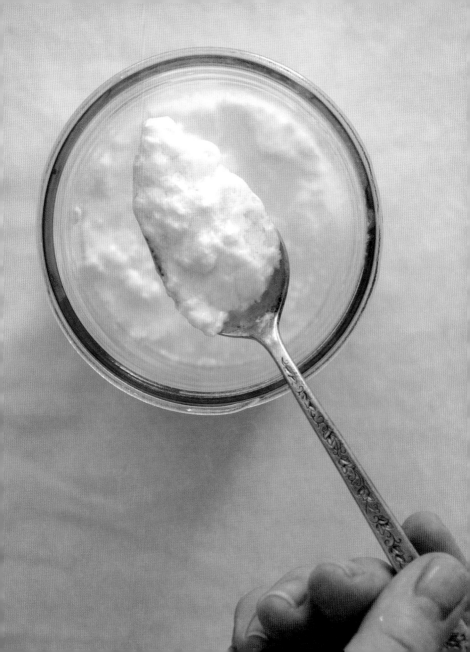

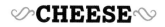

CHEESE

Cheese making is infinite and involves many different variables. Living with goats and abundant milk, my fellow communards and I make cheese frequently.

This is the most basic process for cheese. In its simplest manifestation it is not a fermented food. Aging it will introduce cultures.

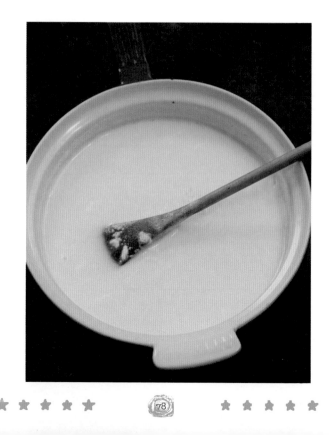

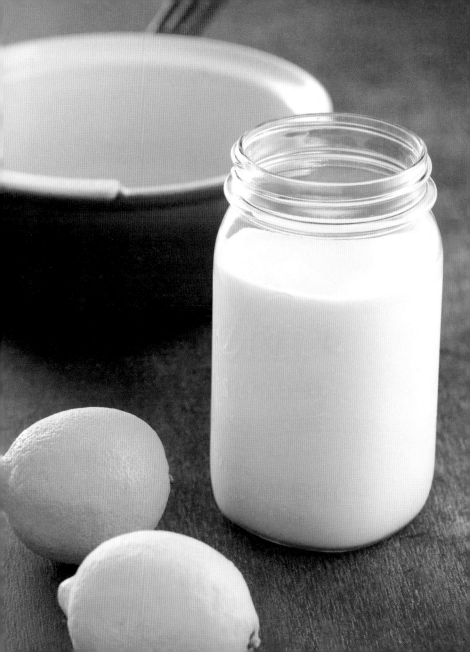

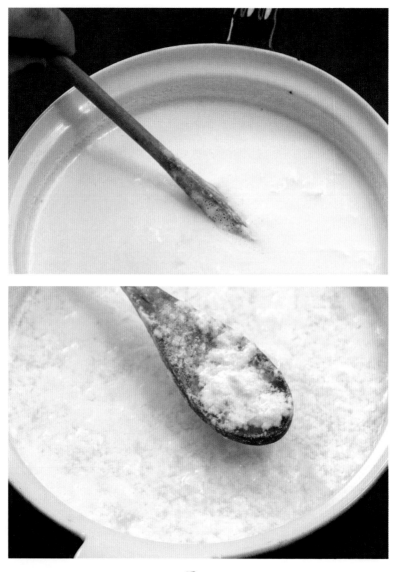

Heat milk to a boil, taking care to stir frequently to avoid burning.

Add some lemon juice and/or vinegar until the milk curdles.

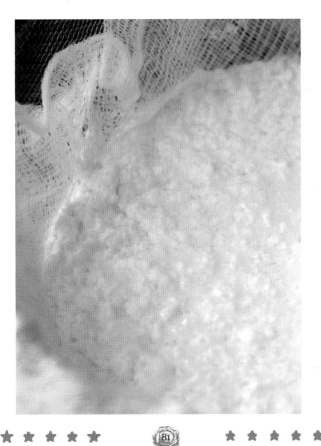

Strain curdled milk through a cheesecloth and squeeze out extra moisture. This is farmers cheese, similar in consistency to ricotta, and great for lasagna or blintzes or Italian-style cheese cake. Taking it a step further will yield the Indian-style cheese paneer:

Place ball of curds in cheesecloth on a sloped surface, like a cutting board with something under one end. Then place a second flat surface on top of the curds, weighted down to *force moisture out.* Leave for a couple of hours or more and when you unwrap the cheesecloth the cheese will hold its form.

Alternatively, you can prepare a ball of cheese to age a bit:
Add salt to strained curds and mix well. The amount of salt will influence the flavor, the consistency and the micro-organism environment of the cheese.

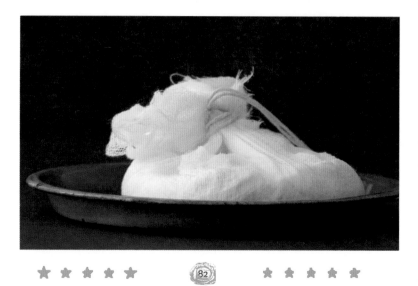

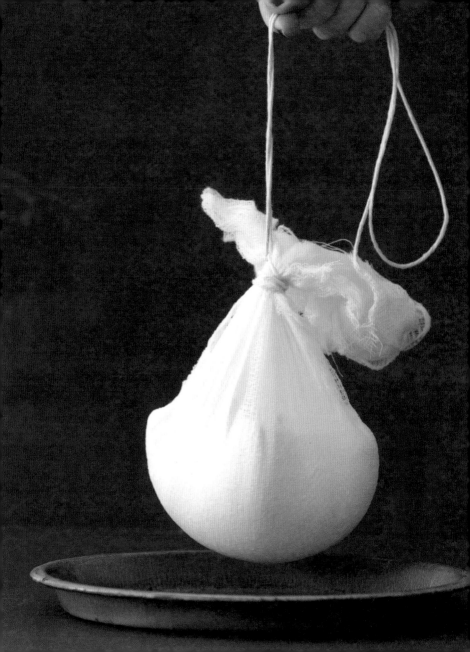

Gather corners of cheesecloth and *let cheese hang in a ball* from a hook or nail, with a bowl underneath to catch dripping liquid.

Eat this after a day or a week or month. Unless you are very systematic about controlling the variables, every cheese will be unique.

Cheese can also be made with rennet, which curdles the cheese at much lower temperatures and produces harder cheeses. Using rennet, you can curdle yogurt or kefir or other cultured milks into cheese without killing the cultures as boiling would. Rennet—from animal or vegetable sources—is available from New England Cheesemaking Supply Company, www.cheesemaking.com, as are many specific cheese cultures.

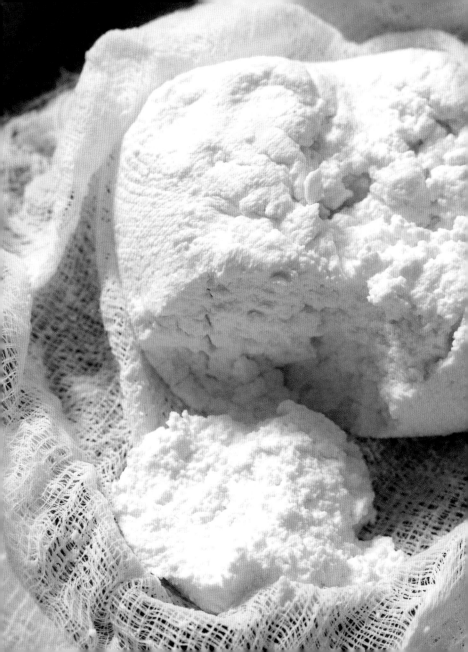

⌒ TEMPEH ⌒

Tempeh is a soybean ferment from Indonesia.

It is worth the trouble of making tempeh yourself. I have nothing against the frozen version available in health food stores, but it is vehicle food—only as good as the flavors you smother it with. Freshly fermented tempeh has a rich, unique, delicious flavor and texture. It involves the most elaborate temperature control of anything in this book, but it is well worth the effort.

Tempeh requires spores of *Rhyzopus oligosporus*. Spores are available inexpensively from:

G.E.M. Cultures
30301 Sherwood Road
Fort Bragg, CA 95437
(707)964-2922
www.gemcultures.com

Tempeh Lab
P.O. Box 208
Summertown, TN 38483
(931)964-3574
TheFarmCommunity.com/
the-tempeh-lab

The Tempeh Lab is located at The Farm, another Tennessee community that was at one time very famous and was instrumental in popularizing tempeh and other soy products in the U.S. *The Farm Vegetarian Cookbook* (information in the bibliography) has excellent detailed tempeh-making directions.

Maintaining a temperature of 85-88 degrees Fahrenheit for 19-26 hours can be tricky. I generally use the oven of our propane stove with just the pilot light on, with a mason jar ring propping the door open enough that

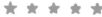

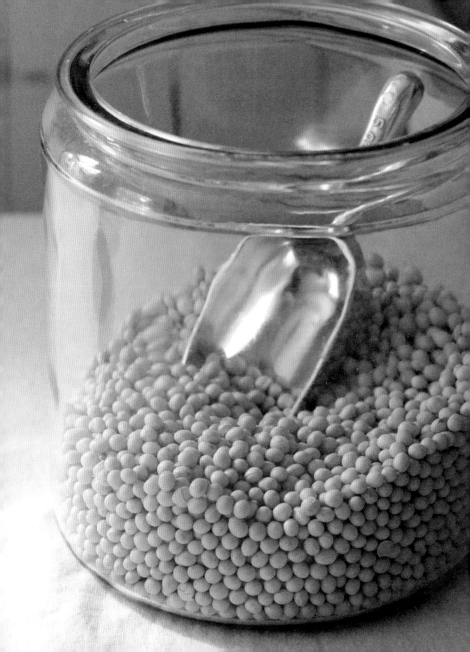

it doesn't get too hot. I also incubated larger quantities of tempeh in the greenhouse on a sunny day, then in a small room somewhat overheated by a wood stove at night. Be sure to maintain good air circulation around the incubating tempeh. Innovate, make it work.

INGREDIENTS *for 8-10 servings:*
2 ½ cups Soybeans
1 teaspoon Spore
2 tablespoons Raw Apple Cider Vinegar

SPECIAL EQUIPMENT:
Clean towels
Zip-lock bags (3 large ones) or a baking tray and aluminum foil

PROCESS:
Crack soybeans in a grain mill, coarsely so that every bean is broken but in just a few large pieces. This helps the beans cook faster and gives more surface area for the spore to grow on. In the absence of a grain grinder you can soak the beans overnight or until they are soft, then roughly chop or food process them. You could also use whole soybeans, or another smaller type of bean.

Boil beans, without salt, until they are soft enough to eat. They do not need to be super soft. The fermentation will soften the beans. As you cook and stir the soybeans, their hulls will rise to the surface of the pot in a foamy froth. Skim off the froth with the hulls and discard.

As the beans boil, take a few zip lock bags and *poke holes* in them with a fork, every couple of inches. The bags provide a form for the tempeh to fill, and the holes assure good air circulation which is necessary for the spore to thrive. You can reuse the bags by cleaning them after use, drying them thoroughly, and storing them in a special place. Alternatively form tempeh in a baking tray with a lip of at least ¾ of an inch, then cover it with foil with fork holes punched every couple of inches.

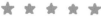

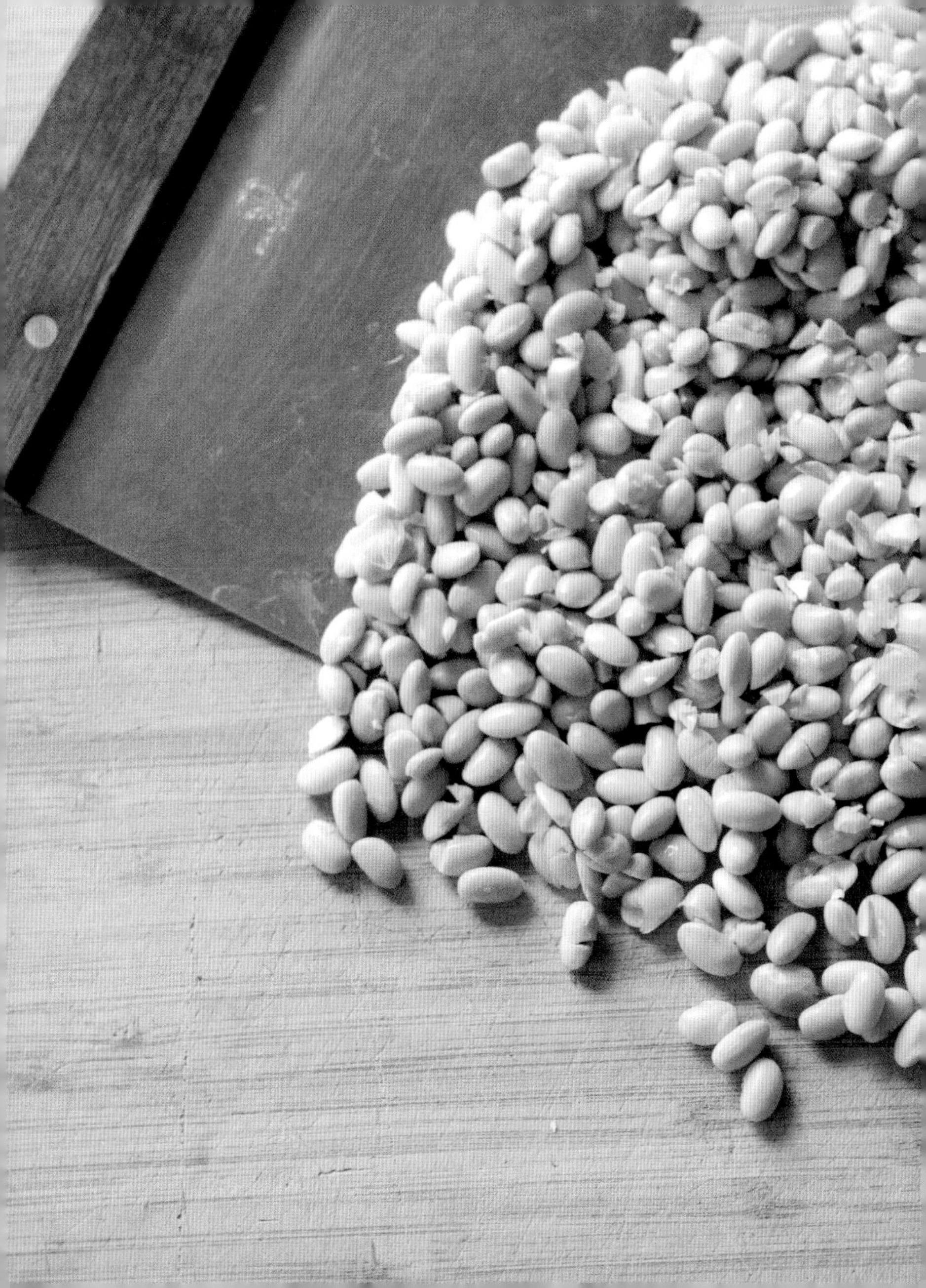

When the beans are ready, strain them and spread them, or a portion of them at a time, on a clean towel. *Use the towel to dry them.* The most common problem with tempeh is excess moisture, which yields a foul inedible product. Swaddle and pat the cooked soybeans until most of the surface moisture has absorbed into the towel. Use a second towel if necessary. It is rare that we have the opportunity to be so intimate with soybeans. Enjoy it.

Place the cooked and dried soybeans in a bowl. *Add vinegar* and mix; *add spore* and mix so the spore is evenly distributed around the soybeans. *Spoon mixture into bags with holes,* spreading it evenly, sealing bags, and placing them on oven racks or wherever they will incubate. Likewise, if you're using a baking pan, spread mixture evenly and cover with foil with holes.

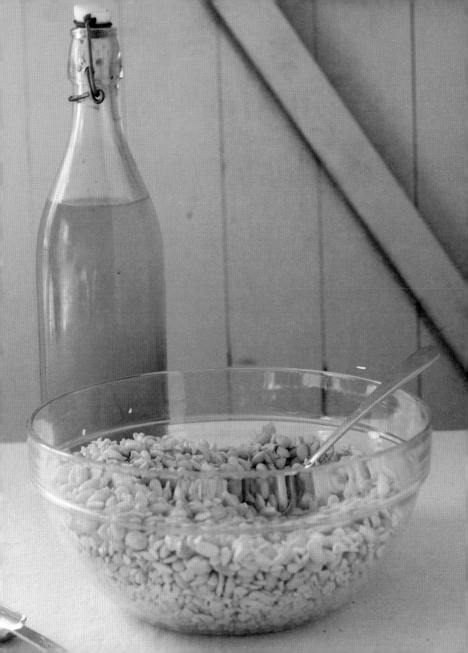

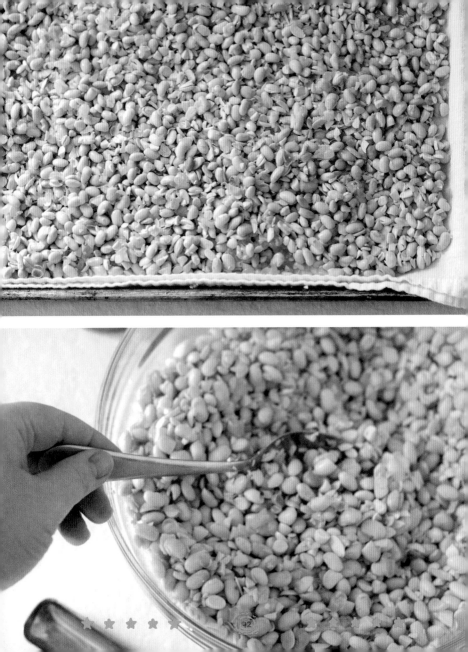

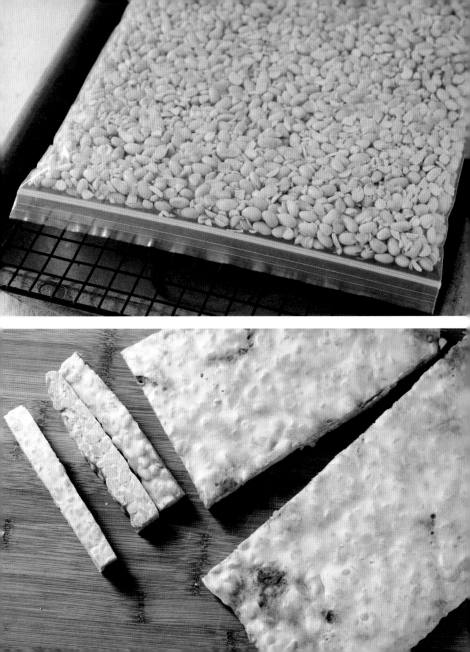

Incubate at about 85-88 degrees fahrenheit for about 19-26 hours.
No dramatic changes occur during the first half of the fermentation period. Start the process in the evening, let it spend the night unattended, then watch the exciting drama of the later period. Hairy white mold begins to form in all the space between soybeans. It begins generating heat, as well, so keep an eye on the temperature and adjust the incubation space as necessary. The mold gradually thickens until it forms a cohesive mat holding the beans together. The tempeh should have a pleasant earthy odor, like button mushrooms or babies. Eventually, the mold will start to show patches of grey or black coloration, originating near the air holes. Once it has large patches of grey or black, it is ready.

Remove tempeh from your incubator and from its forms. Allow it to cool to room temperature before refrigerating. *Tempeh should not be eaten raw.* Sauté slices of it plain to discover its unique flavor. Or prepare it however you like it. You can use grains along with beans in your tempeh. Cook the grain separately, and if you cook it dry there is no need to towel-dry it.

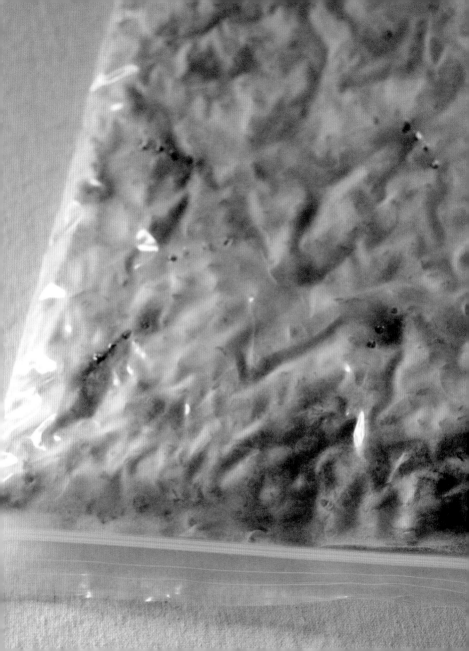

❧TEMPEH REUBENS❧

My favorite way to enjoy tempeh is as a tempeh reuben sandwich.

This sandwich incorporates four different ferments: bread, tempeh, sauerkraut and cheese.

Sauté slices of tempeh in a lightly oiled pan. Spread thousand island dressing (ketchup, mayonnaise, relish) on slices of bread (rye is best). Place sautéed tempeh slices on dressing.

Cover tempeh with a generous portion of sauerkraut. Cover sauerkraut with a thin slice of swiss (or other variety of) cheese. Broil or bake for a minute or so, until cheese is melted. Serve open faced and enjoy.

And how could you eat a reuben sandwich without a pickle?

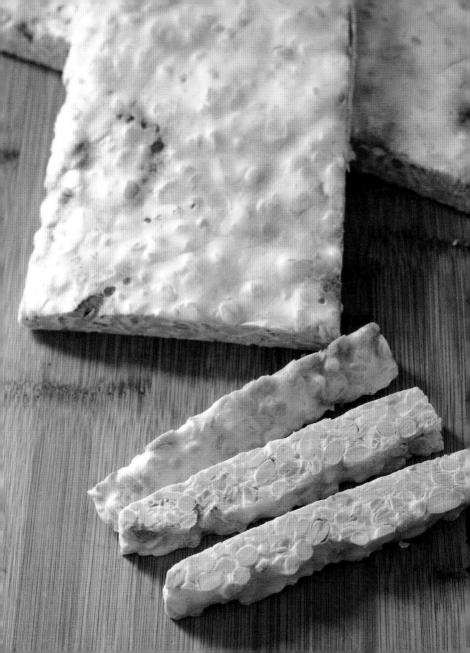

∽BRINE PICKLES∽

Growing up in New York City, I experienced my Jewish heritage largely through food. I developed a taste for sour and half-sour pickles. Most of what is sold in stores as pickles is preserved in vinegar. My idea of a pickle is fermented in a brine solution.

Pickle-making requires close attention. You can't leave it for too many days. My first attempt at brine pickle making resulted in pickles so soft they fell apart. I abandoned it for a few days and perhaps the brine was not salty enough in the heat of the Tennessee summer. "
Our perfection lies in our imperfection." This is one of my mantras and holds true for fermentation. There are, inevitably, a certain number of failed experiments. We are dealing with fickle life forces, after all.

I persevered, compelled by a craving deep inside of me for the yummy garlic dill sour pickles of Gus's pickle stall on the lower east side of Manhattan and Zabar's on the upper west side and Bubbie's in upscale health food stores elsewhere.

One quality prized in a good pickle is crunchiness. Fresh grape leaves are effective at keeping the pickle crunchy. I recommend using them if you have access to some. Also for brine pickle recipes you could use sour cherry leaves, oak leaves, and horseradish leaves.

The biggest variables in pickle-making are cucumber size, brine strength and temperature. I prefer pickles from small and medium cucumbers to pickles from big ones, which can be tough and hollow in the middle. I don't worry about uniformity of size; I just eat the smaller ones first, figuring the larger ones will take longer to ferment. Brine strength is calculated by weight of salt as a percentage of the weight of the solution, and controls the rate of fermentation.

 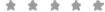

Pickles made in a 10% brine will ferment slowly and last for a long time, but they will taste very salty and require soaking in water to be palatable. Low salt pickles, around 3.5% brine, are half-sours. They ferment fast and don't keep for long. This recipe uses a 5% brine. Temperature, too, factors into the rate of fermentation. If your cucumbers peak when temperatures are in the nineties, you might strengthen your brine a bit to slow things down, and check your pickles daily.

✎ PICKLES ✎

INGREDIENTS *for one gallon:*
Small-medium cucumbers (approximately 4 lbs.)
Salt (3/8 cup)
Fresh flowering dill, or any form of dill (fresh or dried leaf or seeds)
Garlic, lots
Grape leaves (which help cucumbers stay crunchy)
Black peppercorns

SPECIAL EQUIPMENT:
Ceramic crock or food-grade plastic bucket—cylindrical shape
is what's important.
Plate that fits inside crock or bucket.
One gallon jug filled with water, or a big boiled rock.
Cloth cover

PROCESS:
Rinse cucumbers, taking care to not bruise them, and making sure their blossoms end. If you're using cucumbers that aren't fresh off the vine that day, soak them for a couple of hours in very cold water to freshen them.

Boil water, about half a gallon, in which *to dissolve salt*, about 3/8 cup, to create a 5% brine solution. The reason for boiling the water is to make sure all the salt dissolves in the brine solution. Let it cool until it is comfortable to the touch.

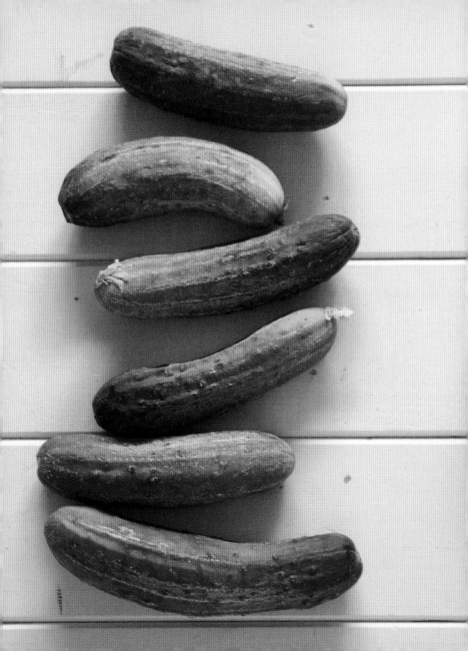

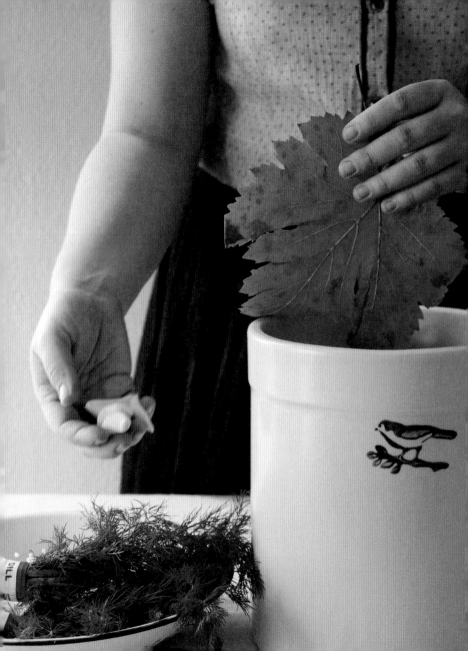

While the brine cools, thoroughly clean the crock, then place at the bottom of it several heads of *dill,* a couple of heads worth of garlic cloves, a pinch of *black peppercorns,* and a handful of fresh *grape leaves.*

Place cucumbers in the crock.

Pour the brine over the cucumbers, place the (clean) plate over them then *weight it down* with a jug filled with water or a boiled rock. If the brine doesn't cover the weighted-down plate, add more brine mixed at the same ratio of 1 tablespoon salt to each cup of water.

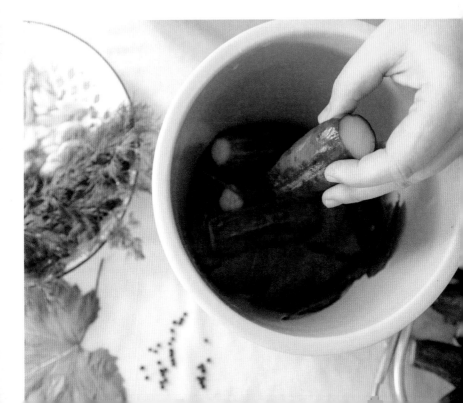

Cover the crock with a cloth to keep out dust and flies and *store it in a cool place. Check the crock every day* and skin any scum from the surface and taste the pickles after a few days.

Enjoy the pickles as they continue to ferment and continue to check the crock every day. Eventually, *after one to four weeks they will be fully sour;* continue to enjoy them, moving them to the fridge to slow down fermentation.

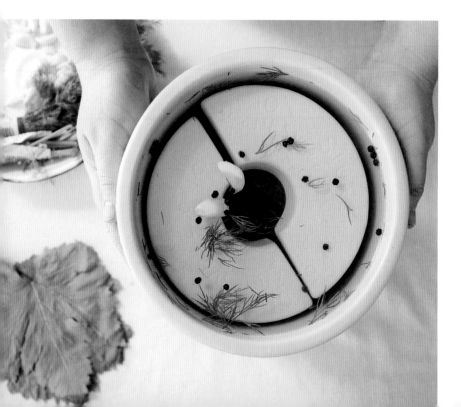

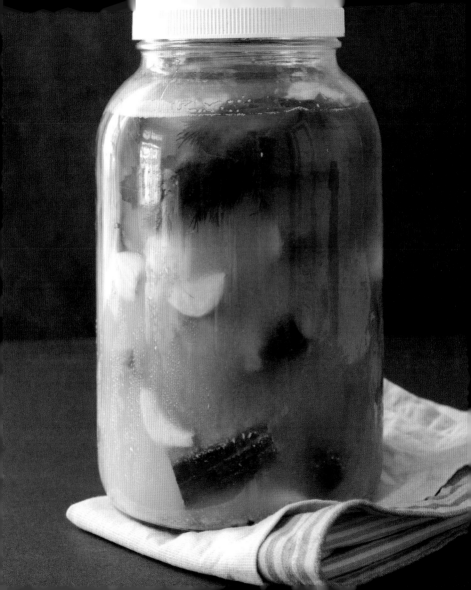

∞CAPERS∞

Capers are their own plant and the delicious savory flavor of commercially-available capers is mostly about the brining process. My friend Lisa Lust and I were eating capers and talking about how much we enjoy them. In food, as in fashion, small accessories make all the difference. Lisa noticed that pods were developing on the abundant milkweed plants and had the idea to try brining them. They are *so* good, better than capers from the store, I daresay. And made from a weed that seems to grow everywhere.

INGREDIENTS *(makes one quart)*:
Milkweed pods, almost a quart's worth
Salt
Garlic.

PROCESS:
Pick milkweed pods. Pods appear after the big flowers fall away. Try to catch them when they are small. *Boil water*, about 2 cups, and *dissolve salt,* about 2 tablespoons, in it to create a brine solution.

Let it cool until comfortable to the touch.

Fill a quart jar with milkweed pods and garlic, a head's worth of peeled cloves or as much as you have patience to peel. *Pour the cooled brine over the pods* to cover them. If you don't have enough brine, add a little more water and salt.

Weigh down the pods in the brine.
We used a smaller jar that fit inside the mouth of the jar that contained the pods and brine. Improvise.
The important thing is to keep the pods under the protection of the brine.

Taste the capers daily. Ours tasted good but not quite ripe after about four days. After a week, a film of scum appeared on the surface. I skimmed it off, tasted the capers, and they were perfect. **Keep in refrigerator** and use as needed.

✒KIMCHI✒

Kimchi is another brine ferment that I have loved for years. It is a Korean pickle made in many different styles. In certain respects, Kimchi is like sauerkraut. One difference is that kimchi recipes generally call for heavily salting the cabbage to soften it quickly, then rinsing it and fermenting it with less salt. Kimchi is also spicy, using generous amounts of ginger, garlic and hot chili peppers. Kimchi ferments faster than sauerkraut. You could certainly make it in a crock like sauerkraut, but this recipe is for a small quantity using a quart-size jar.

INGREDIENTS *for one quart of kimchi:*
1 large head chinese cabbage (nappa or bok choi)
Sea Salt
1 small daikon radish
a few green onions (including tops)
a few cloves of garlic
1 or 2 hot red chilies, depending on how hot peppery you like food
2 teaspoons fresh ginger

PROCESS:
Mix a brine of about four cups of water and 2 tablespoons of salt.
Coarsely chop the cabbage and let it soak in the brine until soft,
a few hours or overnight.

Prepare other ingredients: slice radish and green onions into thin strips; grate the ginger; finely chop the garlic and chili and mix it into a paste with the ginger.

Remove the cabbage from the brine and rinse it well, with several changes of water.

 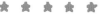

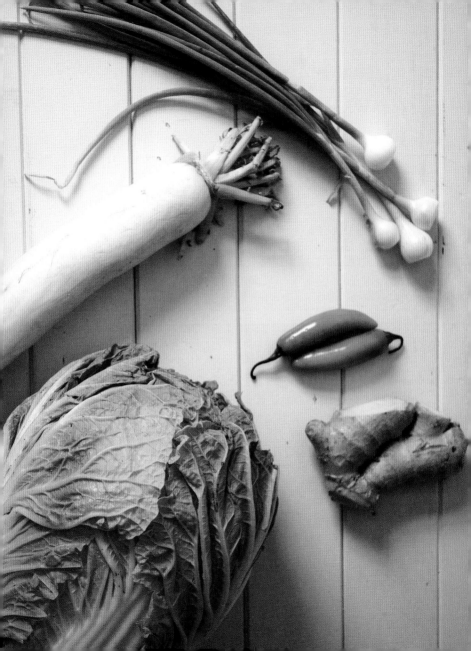

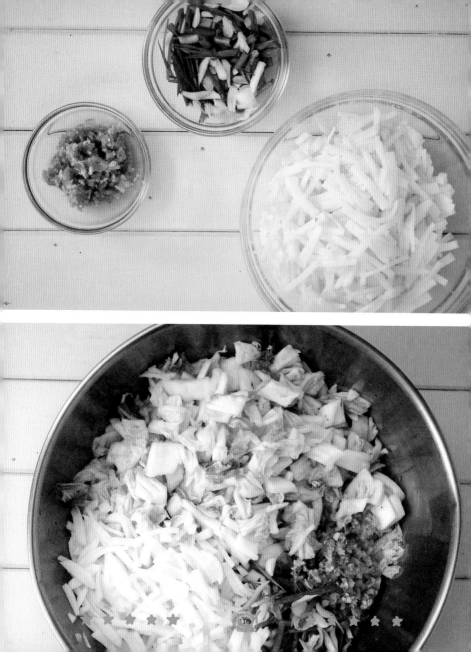

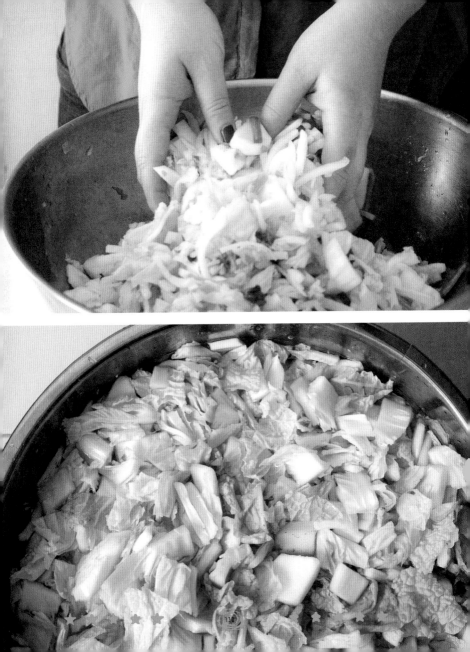

Mix the cabbage with the radish and onion strips, sprinkle the vegetables with about one tablespoon of salt, and add the garlic-ginger-chili paste.

Mix everything together thoroughly and stuff into clean quart-size jar. Add enough water to submerge the vegetables and cover the jar (not tightly).

Taste the kimchi every day. After several days of fermentation, when it tastes ripe, move it to the refrigerator to slow down the process.

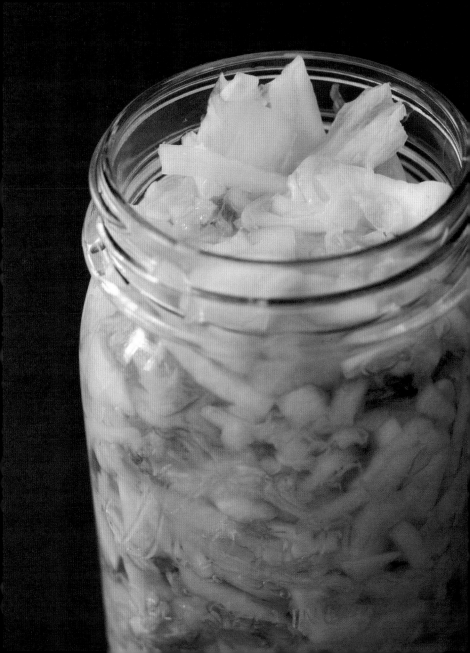

❧ A NOTE ON CHOCOLATE ❧

I was excited to learn that cocoa beans go through a fermentation process between harvest and roasting to develop the flavor and qualities that satisfy us deeply. But I have no easy home recipe to impart.

Though I love chocolate, both eating it and cooking with it, I've never had the opportunity to participate in the basic underlying transformative processes which create chocolate from cocoa beans. Interestingly, during my African travels a decade and a half ago, I met cocoa farmers who had never eaten chocolate. Growers and consumers of this luscious confection are isolated from the transformative process. It's a classic scenario of alienated labor and consumption in the global village. I'm ready for the D.I.Y. cocoa bean to chocolate truffle workshop. Just tell me when and where.

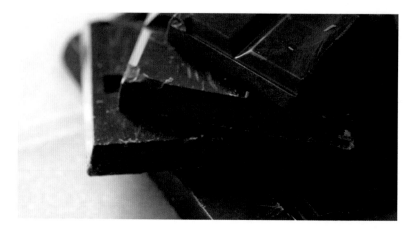

⭐ ⭐ ⭐ ⭐ ⭐ ⭐ ⭐ ⭐ ⭐ ⭐

∽A NOTE ON COMPOST∽

Today I used some of my compost tea in the garden. It is a garbage barrel full of horse manure and seaweed and comfrey leaves and dead fish and water, bubbling away. I dilute the tea with water and use it to feed plants. Fresh from drinking kefir and eating sauerkraut and feeding my sourdough, I was struck by how similar the compost tea is to all these other bubbling brews, so full of life and deep nourishment. And indeed, it too is a fermentation process, another slice of the dance of life and decay.

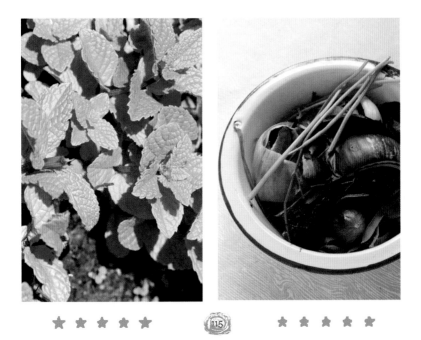

✥AGITATION✥
A POLITICAL NOTE

The word fermentation has another connotation. Ideas ferment, as they spread and mutate and inspire movements for change. In the American Heritage dictionary the secondary meaning of fermentation is "unrest, agitation." I feel equally committed to this aspect of fermentation.

As an agent for change, I am a culturural manipulator, proud to be subversive.

As you watch your fermenting food bubble away as bacteria and yeast work their transformative magic, envision yourself as an agent for change, creating agitation and unrest, releasing bubbles of transformation into the social order. Use your fermented goodies to nourish your family and friends and allies. The life-affirming power of these basic foods contrasts sharply with the lifeless industrially-processed foods that fill supermarket shelves.

Draw inspiration from the action of bacteria and yeast, and make your life a transformative process.

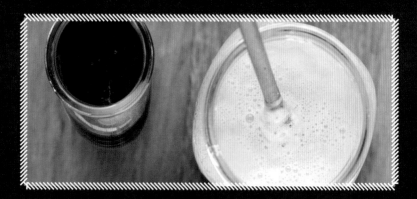

✐ANNOTATION✐
A HISTORICAL NOTE

I am writing this in Bowdoinham, Maine, at the home of my friend Ed Curran and his kids Caity and Roman. Sometimes I need breaks from the intensity of community living, and I am grateful to them for sharing their home with me and my bubbling jars and crocks. As I wrote and talked about the project, Ed's father Bob, who is an avid collector of all sorts of random stuff, especially books, brought me volume 9 ("Extraction to Gambrinus") of the 1944 *Encyclopedia Britannica*, which contains an extensive article on fermentation. The article, in the smug definitive tone of that authoritative reference work, provides a sort of intellectual history of the shifting human perceptions of the transformative processes we call fermentation, which are believed to have been enjoyed by humans for at least 8,000 years. Following are some particularly informative and/or poetic passages from this lengthy article.

> "Yeast is now known to be a living material, and the spores or germs of yeast are to be found everywhere adherent to the particles of dust in the air. Consequently any sugary material exposed to the air quickly becomes fermented. Prior to the discovery of such germs in the atmosphere the ferment or leaven was supposed either to have been produced spontaneously, generated as it were, within the material itself by some occult force, or else to have been derived from pre-existing yeast from time immemorial. This latter view was nearer the truth, for it conceived of yeast as something akin to life. Indeed when questioned as to the origins of the Kephir ferment, which is analogous to yeast, Mohammedans in the Caucasus to this day will declare that the first grains of Kephir were put there by Allah. And is not, in the New Testament, the comparison of the Kingdom of Heaven, made at one time to a seed, and at another time to leaven? It would be fallacious, therefore, to imagine because of the materialistic tendencies of the alchemists, that humanity had never had any conception of yeast as a living thing, or of fermentation as a process akin to life..."

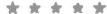

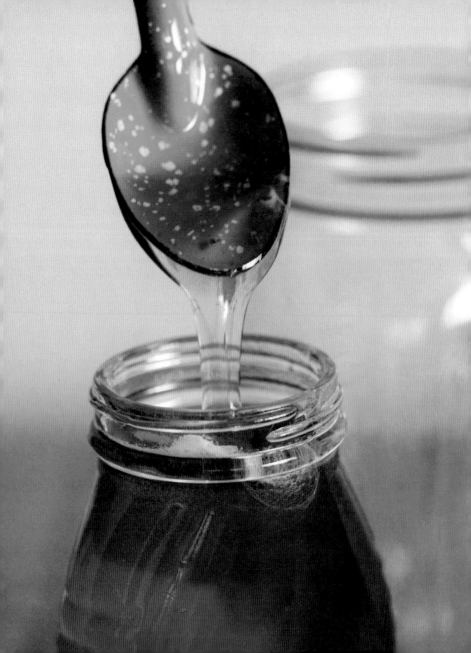

"It is impossible to place any date to the antiquity of the art of fermentation, and much that passes at the present time as novel was known to the ancients..."

"Such ancient practices, however, hardly found any echo in the ideas of the 18th and early 19th century. Vitalism was in disrepute, the microscope had not been perfected, and its revelations were but little credited; chemistry had just made rapid strides to the front, and organic chemistry...had become established as the sure way to a study of physiology, medicine and agriculture. Any attempt to introduce vague and unknown causes, as for examples a possible influence of microscopic forms of life in the process of fermentation, was considered retrograde and branded as vitalistic..."

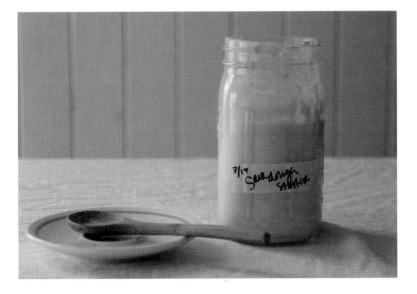

"Louis Pasteur opened the eyes of mankind to a new world of microscopic life...Each type of fermentation was shown to be correlated with the life of some special microscopic organism, multiplying with incredible velocity. Fermentation, putrefaction and the slow process of combustion by which dead organic matter is resolved into mineral matter, at that time designated spontaneous combustion, were all shown to be caused by the agency of microbes, and to cease when the life was destroyed..."

"Fermentation has, in common parlance, come to have two meanings; on the one hand it refers to alcoholic fermentation, which on account of its great industrial importance, overshadows all other types of fermentation: and, on the other hand, it refers to a large variety of changes which occur in connection with animal and plant life...Academically speaking, however, these phenomenon all come under one head. Ambiguity will be avoided if we use the word fermentation to describe the whole process set up by the living cells, the growth and multiplication of the cells, as well as the decomposition set up in the medium by their agency either in, around or outside the cells, while we reserve the word enzyme action to describe the individual fermentative acts, when disassociated from the living organism, or considered, even for purposes of discussion, as acting independently of the life of the cell..."

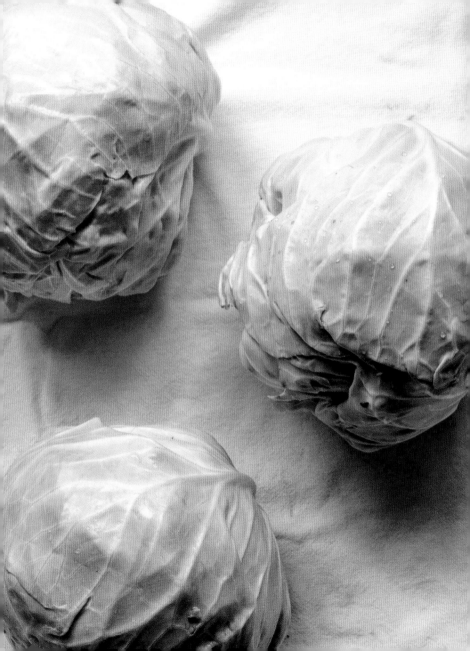

✑INFORMATION✑

A BIBLIOGRAPHICAL NOTE

Sandor Ellix Katz, *Wild Fermentation: The Flavor, Nutrition, and Craft of Live-Culture Foods* (Chelsea Green, 2003, 2016). The follow-up book to this one.

Sandor Ellix Katz, *The Revolution Will Not Be Microwaved* (Chelsea Green, 2006). An exploration of alternative food ideas and movements.

Sandor Ellix Katz, *The Art of Fermentation* (Chelsea Green, 2012) More than ten years into learning about fermentation, this book further expands on ever-developing ideas.

Stephen Harrod Buhner, *Sacred and Healing Beers: The Secrets of Ancient Fermentation*, Siris Books, 1998. A very different home brew book with lots of information and lore and simple down-to-earth processes.

Louise Hagler and Dorothy R. Bates, editors, *The New Farm Vegetarian Cookbook,* Book Publishing Co., 1989. The most detailed tempeh instructions around, with good photos and troubleshooting help. Lots of other classic veggie recipes, too.

Aveline Kushi, *Aveline Kushi's Complete Guide to Macrobiotic Cooking*, Warner Books, 1989. The wife of macrobiotics guru Michio Kushi offers many simple Japanese brine pickling techniques.

★ ★ ★ ★ ★   122   ★ ★ ★ ★ ★

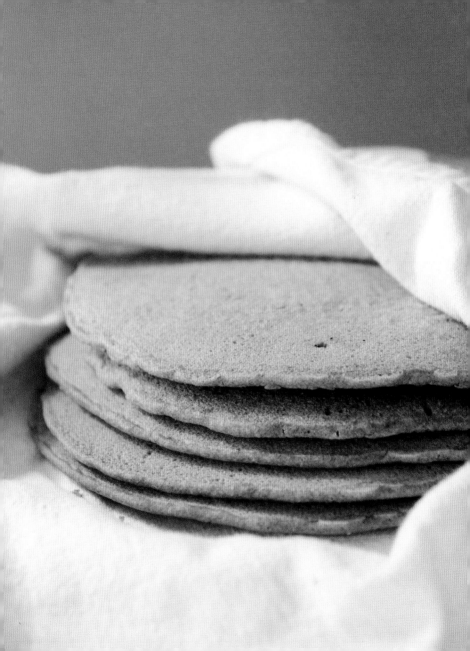

Daniel and Judith Blahnik, *Bread Alone: Bold Fresh Loaves From Your Own Hands*, William Morrow & Co., 1993. Really good sourdough bread making techniques, in excruciating detail, with lots of ideas for variations.

Bill Mollison, *The Permaculture Book of Ferment and Human Nutrition*, Tagari Publications, 1993. An encyclopedic survey of fermentation and other food preservation and transformation techniques around the globe, by the founder and guru of "permaculture." This is the fermentation freak's bible.

William Shurtleff and Akiko Aoyagi, *The Book of Miso*, Ballantine, 1981. This book has recipes for many varieties of miso, instructions for making your own koji, and more information, recipe ideas and folklore about miso than you ever imagined.

Laura Ziedrich, *The Joy of Pickling*, The Harvard Common Press, 1998. This book has great detailed information on brine pickling, Sauerkraut, kimchi and many other variations, including helpful troubleshooting guides.

I've included sources I use for obtaining specific cultures with the recipes that call for them. To obtain other cultures you may wish to investigate in your fermentation adventures, these are the best all-around sources:

CulturesForHealth.com
Yemoos.com

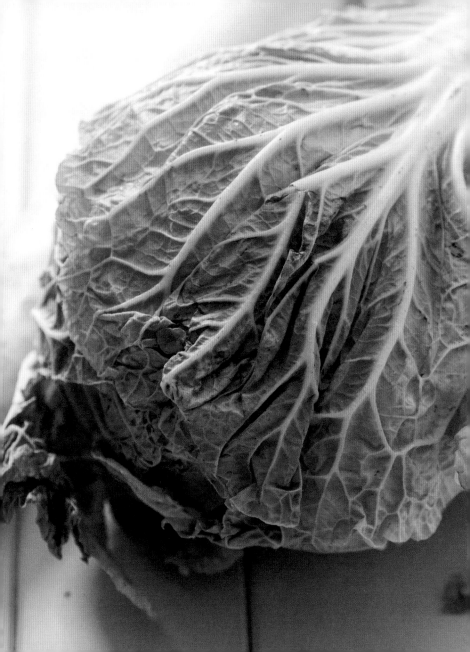

✑ ABOUT THE AUTHOR ✑

Sandor Ellix Katz is a *New York Times* best-selling author and fermentation revivalist. His interest in fermentation grew out of overlapping interests in cooking, nutrition and gardening. After writing this book in 2001, he was inspired to write a longer version, *Wild Fermentation: The Flavor, Nutrition, and Craft of Live-Culture Foods* (Chelsea Green, 2003). That and his subsequent books *The Revolution Will Not Be Microwaved* (Chelsea Green, 2006) and *The Art of Fermentation* (Chelsea Green, 2012), along with the hundreds of fermentation workshops he has taught around the world, have helped to catalyze a broad revival of the fermentation arts. A self-taught experimentalist who lives in rural Tennessee, the *New York Times* calls him "one of the unlikely rock stars of the American food scene." Sandor is the recipient of a James Beard award and many other honors.

For more information, check out his website WildFermentation.com.

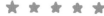

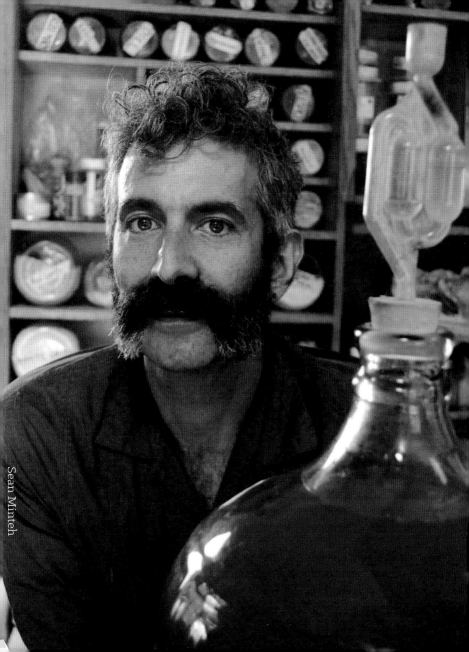

SUBSCRIBE TO EVERYTHING WE PUBLISH!

Do you love what Microcosm publishes?

Do you want us to publish more great stuff?

Would you like to receive each new title as it's published?

Subscribe as a BFF to our new titles and we'll mail them all to you as they are released!

$10-30/mo, pay what you can afford. Include your t-shirt size and your birthday for a possible surprise!

microcosmpublishing.com/bff

...AND HELP US GROW YOUR SMALL WORLD!

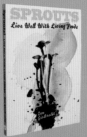
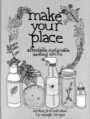
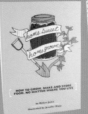
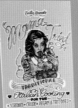
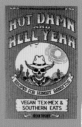